HERE IS WHAT THEY ARE SAYING:

"Thanks for saving my sex life." — *J.E. (Post-Partum Pelvic Pain)*

"*Ending Female Pain* is a treasure. Isa Herrera has put together the best possible resource for helping women heal pelvic pain and live fully and comfortably."
> — *Christiane Northrup, MD, ob/gyn physician and author of the New York Times bestsellers: Women's Bodies, Women's Wisdom and The Wisdom of Menopause*

"My patients recover faster and have less pain after doing Isa's exercises and receiving her unique treatments. Hands-down she is the best in NYC."
> — *Jacques Moritz, MD, Director, Division of Gynecology, St. Luke's Roosevelt Hospital*

"A breakthrough for women... this book is the ultimate self-healing resource for chronic pelvic pain and post-partum complications."
> — *Ricki Lake and Abby Epstein, filmmakers of The Business of Being Born and authors of Your Best Birth*

"Before I started doing Isa's exercises the pain was so severe I couldn't even sit."
> — *D.P. NYC (Interstitial Cystitis and Pelvic Pain)*

"The homework, exercises and treatment that Isa gave me helped me. Today I am pain free." — *K.J.C. (Pelvic Pain)*

"Isa proved to be my secret weapon against vestibulodynia. She has made it her life's work to understand how to unlock the body to lessen the grip of vaginal pain. Isa got me ready both physically and psychologically to face the frightening realities of a vestibulectomy. Whenever I would get discouraged, she would help me build up my mental framework and shore me up against the frustrations of this very mentally-challenging disease."
> — *J. Q. (Vestibulitis and Post-Surgical Vestibulectomy Patient)*

Published in the United States by Duplex Publishing, New York.

2nd Edition, 1st Printing, April 2014

10 Digit ISBN: 0615988636

13 Digit EAN: 978-0615988634 (Duplex Publishing)

Medical Disclaimer:

Consult and seek the advice of your Doctor and/or Physical Therapist before attempting these exercises or self-help tools found in *Ending Female Pain*. The medical information in this book is provided for informational purposes only, and is not to be used or relied on for any diagnostic or treatment purposes. This information is intended to be educational only and does not create any patient-physical therapist relationship, and should not be used as a substitute for professional diagnosis and treatment. Serious injury could result from improper performance of these techniques and exercises. If pain occurs with any exercise STOP immediately. Neither Renew Physical Therapy, PC, nor Isa Herrera, MSPT, CSCS, can be held liable for injury caused by the improper performance of these exercises or self-help tools. The self-help tips found in this book are merely a guide; this book is not intended as a prescription for Physical Therapy. To prevent injury seek the advice of your Doctor or Physical Therapist before attempting any exercise, self-help tip or implementation of any of the information in this book.

Most patients need a multi-layered approach to overcome their chronic pelvic pain. Make sure to see doctors and specialists in the field of female sexual pain and pelvic floor muscle dysfunction, and then talk to your doctor about getting a referral to a physical therapist that specializes in pelvic floor muscle dysfunction. It is also extremely important to educate yourself about your pelvic pain condition. Do not be afraid to ask questions of your caregivers, or to get a second opinion about your condition.

ENDING
female
PAIN

A Woman's Manual

*The Ultimate Self-Help Guide for Women
Suffering from Chronic Pelvic and Sexual Pain*

ISA HERRERA
MSPT, CSCS

2nd Edition

Dedications

For my husband, David, and daughter, Ella.
You are the springboards that allow me to fly.
You are the skeletons of my soul.
You are winds behind me and the love that engulfs me.
You make my spirit soar and my heart sing the song of joy.
I can never repay you for the way you hold space
for me so that I can realize my dreams.
You are the sculptors of my life.

For Stuart Black,
Who helped awaken the healer within me.
You taught me how to search for the truth
with love, compassion, and forgiveness.
I will always be grateful to you.

For my female patients,
who motivate me to think outside the box
to fine-tune the tools and mind-body techniques in this book.
Their stories and firm resolve to end their pain continue
to fuel my search for answers.

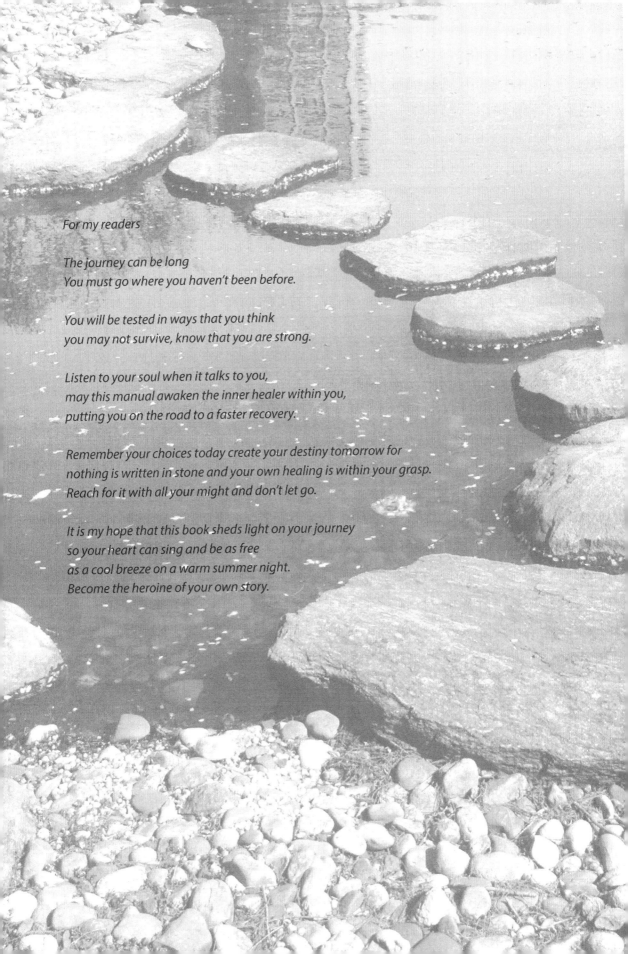

For my readers

The journey can be long
You must go where you haven't been before.

You will be tested in ways that you think
you may not survive, know that you are strong.

Listen to your soul when it talks to you,
may this manual awaken the inner healer within you,
putting you on the road to a faster recovery.

Remember your choices today create your destiny tomorrow for
nothing is written in stone and your own healing is within your grasp.
Reach for it with all your might and don't let go.

It is my hope that this book sheds light on your journey
so your heart can sing and be as free
as a cool breeze on a warm summer night.
Become the heroine of your own story.

Acknowledgements

David Ondrick
Digital Production, Project Management and Editing
A big heartfelt thanks for your vision. You are an extraordinary man who does what needs to be done without hesitation and with vigor and determination.

Betsy Gonzalez & Rachel Schneiderman
Thank you for being there for me in ways that allow me to do the work that I promised I would do. You keep me on track.

To my Renew Physical Therapy Team
For your endless support. You guys rock.
Without you we would not be able to help the many who come to our doors for help. My hat goes off to you guys and my heart sings to have you as part of my team.

Maria Paz Cabardo, Design
You are a visionary designer and overall beautiful person.

Nancie Salicrup
You are a make-up artist extraordinaire!

Richard Simpson, Photographer
Thank you for taking the photos. You always astonish me. You are one creative soul.

Dr. Jacques Moritz
For his insightful foreword and support. Your dedication to the work of helping women always amazes me.

Marissa Klapwald, Main Editor, Elizabeth Ellis, Book Production
For great insights and quick turnaround on the editing and production.

Solange Ross, Model & Women's Health Physical Therapist
Thank you being part of this project. You did it with grace.

Collin Pisarra & Winston Johnson, Digital Photos and Illustrations
Thank you for being flexible and getting the work done. Your easy nature makes working with you guys a joy.

Rosita Arvigo, Kathe Wallace, Holly Herman, Elizabeth Noble, Dr. Elaine Rosen, and Dr. Martha Sliwinski for inspiring me to be the best; Amy Slotnick for guidance and direction, my mom Crucita for being mom; and Ricki Lake and Abby Epstein for helping increase awareness on the topic of women's health.

ENDING female PAIN

A Woman's Manual

2nd Edition

Contents

Contents Continued

Appendices

Foreword

by Dr. Jacques Moritz

Director of Obstetrics and Gynecology Division, St. Luke's Roosevelt Hospital

In my over 15 years of work at St. Luke's, I have seen women from all walks of life who experience sexual pain or some other type of pelvic disorder. More often than not, these women end up suffering quietly because they are told that the pain is in their heads. They quickly give up, unaware that there are remedies to get them back to normal.

Doctors are often ignorant of these remedies because they are not trained in medical school in ways to deal with post-operative, post-delivery or generalized vulvar pain, much less pain during sexual intercourse. Sadly, many women are also brought up to accept pelvic pain as part of their lives.

Although pelvic health and rehabilitation is a critical part of female wellness, it is often the most neglected aspect of their care in this country. I believe the main reason for this neglect is because no one wants to deal with or talk about pain in a woman's vagina. After a woman has a baby, a pelvic surgery, or experiences painful intercourse, often no effort is made to eliminate the pain or to test whether her pelvic floor muscles function properly. In other countries like France, for example, pelvic rehabilitation is considered an integral part of the healing process post-childbirth and pelvic surgery. It only makes sense to treat trauma to a very delicate area the same way a broken leg requires therapy.

The first thing women need to know is that the pain is not in their heads. Pelvic pain is not a normal part of life, that sex is supposed to be pleasurable, and if there is pain, it is a sign that something is wrong. If your current doctor does not believe in this philosophy there are three things you can do to help yourself. One, find a doctor that understands this philosophy. Two, while your doctor understands this philosophy, you also need to understand that pelvic pain is a source of frustration to them because they are not trained to deal with this. Three, seek out a physical therapist who specializes in pelvic floor muscle rehabilitation. In the United States, doctors do not routinely recommend this type of rehabilitation, causing women to suffer needlessly. That is why this book is so important for women everywhere.

It must also be known that there are no quick fixes for pelvic pain; there isn't a cream, gel, or an exercise that is going to fix it. It is going to be a series of trials and errors but it can be done. Frustration will make the situation worse than when it started. Isa has taken an interest where most physical therapists do not even want to deal with – a field that most find is not for them. She listens to women, is responsive, understands their pain, and does everything in her power to rehabilitate them. She is also realistic and understands her patients are not always going to end up with zero pain, but she always tries everything in her arsenal of tools to help women avoid unnecessary surgeries.

Ending Female Pain is the most complete resource on the market that offers women self-help treatment from pains caused by childbirth trauma, scar pains from abdominal surgeries, and chronic pelvic and sexual pain, empowering them to overcome their pain themselves. Isa has a unique talent. She is very committed to teaching her patients to break their cycles of pain, whether psychologically or with physical therapy, or both. She believes that hope of recovery lies with her patients and puts them on the path to getting better themselves. In *Ending Female Pain,* Isa gives you the proven strategies and unique techniques that have brought relief to countless numbers of her patients – precisely the information that women need to restore their sexual and day-to-day function, and that is why I highly recommend this book.

Author's Preface to the 2nd Edition

It's been nearly five years since the first printing of *Ending Female Pain*. First and foremost, I would like to thank all my readers for their generous support and reviews of the book. I always intended for *Ending Female Pain* to be a self-help manual focused on awakening the healer within you, but it has also become a resource used by clinicians. The positive response to the book has shown me that there is a great need for the information and advice I can provide. There is so much I want to say about pelvic floor physical therapy that I was compelled to revise the book with relevant updates and additions.

I wrote this second edition of *Ending Female Pain* to further my philosophy that every woman holds the key to her health and well-being. *Ending Female Pain, 2nd Edition* is designed not only to give women better and more powerful pain-relieving tools, but also to help them see that they really can manage their symptoms and pain on their own with the proper direction.

This is not conventional therapy, and it works best when women remain open to treating the whole person. While adding to the already solid foundation of the earlier book, *Ending Female Pain, 2nd Edition* will simultaneously open your mind and dispel fear about the possibility of doing different types of exercises and techniques on yourself. By taking care of your mind, body and soul, you will triumph and get back the life that pain has stolen from you.

In this new and exciting second edition I have added new chapters covering the following: demystifying pudendal nerve neuralagia; coccydynia; the real deal for bladder healing; the clearest and most intelligently effective core training; and an updated external trigger point therapy chapter that paves the way to the restoration of your female power.

The updated chapter, "Decreasing Pelvic Floor Pain with External Hands-On Techniques," includes new external tools that women can use as part of their healing program—all of which I teach my patients here at Renew PT. This chapter now provides a more detailed road map to finding trigger points in different areas of the body that can be contributing to your pelvic pain. Based both on my clinical experience and on science, I believe you will have much success with your therapy when you incorporate these new tools into your self-healing program.

In the new chapter titled "The New Core for Female Pelvic Power," I seek to once and for all dispel the high level of confusion among pelvic sufferers about their abdominal workouts. All over the Internet and in many books abdominal training is discouraged when you suffer from pelvic pain. I have created a new workout for the core that redefines what it means to train the core properly and in synchronization with the pelvic floor muscles. This new chapter focuses on working the innermost transverse abdominal muscle. This is the key that will help restore your female power back to its glory without creating more pain and dysfunction in the pelvic floor muscles.

I've included discussions of pudendal nerve neuralgia and coccydynia in this book because many of the women I treat suffering from these conditions are distraught, and don't know how to find pain relief. Along with the rest of the book these two new chapters take you on a journey of anatomy, self-healing exercises and hands-on tools that will help you manage pain related to these two conditions.

This second edition is intended as an enlightening source of information that adds to what you have been offered in the first book. But keep in mind that it is up to you to make the program work for you. Your road to healing will require commitment and a readiness to make the following promises:

The *Ending Female Pain*, 2nd Edition Requirements:

1. Open-mindedness and a strong intent to get the work done that is required of you.
2. Renunciation of negative self-talk, negative thinking and catastrophic thinking.
3. Sacrifice of your time. You will need to work within this program in the beginning one hour per day.
4. You must have an internal desire to get better. The healing process takes time and you may experience setbacks.
5. A commitment to stay in the present moment without projecting into the future or the past.
6. An understanding on your part that there is no cookie-cutter approach to this program. You must experiment with all the tools and discover what exercises or techniques work best for you.
7. Patience with yourself and the ability to learn all the tools in this second edition. You will need to practice many times to master the techniques and exercises in this book.
8. You must have focused attention when working on yourself using the tools highlighted in this second edition. If you don't, you risk hurting or injuring yourself.
9. You must listen to your body; never override a pain signal or a voice in your head that tells you something is wrong. It could save you from a flare-up or more pain.
10. Fearlessness. You must be fearless and understand you are not alone. Always remind yourself you are a fearless warrior. Don't let fear stop you from achieving your goals and getting your life back.

_____

Your signature here

I have read the above requirements and I understand what it will take to heal.
This signature serves as a contract between my inner healer and me.
I understand that I alone hold the key to my healing.

Now that you understand what is required of you, read *Ending Female Pain, 2nd Edition* and make yourself the heroine of your own story.

Part 1
OVERVIEW

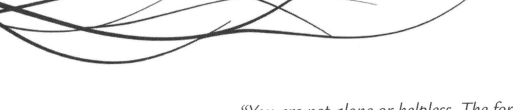

*"You are not alone or helpless. The force
that guides the stars guides you too."*
*– Shrii Shrii
Anandamurti*

Chapter 1

INTRODUCTION

How does one get involved in my line of work? This is a question I am often asked by my patients. As I have come to realize, I always knew I wanted to be involved with women's health. My experiences in the last ten years – first as a fitness instructor and now as a physiotherapist - have shaped my vision of care and empowerment. After hearing the stories of my patients, I have decided to write a self-help manual for the relief of sexual pain based on the various treatments I have given them.

My first exposure to pelvic floor muscle dysfunction came when I taught pre- and post-natal exercise classes in New York City. I was always interested in the things my students told me about the pain they were feeling. Hearing the things these women had to say and what they were going through piqued my interest, but as a pre- and post-natal fitness instructor I lacked the tools and knowledge to help these women on such a complex level. They would tell me things like, "After I had my baby it hurts every time I have sex"; "After the baby came, my husband no longer fits inside me"; "My episiotomy scar opens up after sex"; or "I've never been comfortable having sex at all." I am here to tell you not to be afraid to talk about these issues, because they are common threads among women I have treated and are not spoken about freely enough in the community.

I know now that these problems can be grouped under blanket terms like vulvodynia, dyspareunia, vaginismus, and perineal pain. Many of their complaints are related to pelvic floor muscle (PFM) dysfunctions such as incoordination, spasms, muscle hypertonicity, muscle shortness, trigger points and scar adhesions. Hearing their stories and trying to answer their questions about why they were in pain inspired me to embark on a quest for answers to end female pain. After the birth of my own child, things just didn't feel right down there. And then after a yeast infection and several bouts of antibiotics, not only did sex hurt but now my vulva would burn with a constant ache. After my own personal experience with sexual pain, and after hearing countless stories of other women's bouts with chronic pelvic pain, I decided to make it my life's mission to help women heal their pelvic pain conditions.

At first I found no single resource out there to free myself from vaginal discomfort and pain, so I started to educate myself on PFM dysfunction. I studied with the best teachers, shadowed many doctors in their practices, took countless courses on the topic of PFM dysfunction, and finished my Masters in Physical Therapy. I decided that the best way to help my patients was to create a central source from which they could identify their conditions and empower themselves to overcome their pain. After several years of toil, I was able to open my own healing center in New York City, which I call Renew Physical Therapy.

At my healing center, I give the women under my care many different tools, exercises and techniques to use at home, which I collectively call "The Renew Program for Women™." Many find complete relief with my treatments and unique protocols, and some experience life-changing relief from their chronic pain. To see what some of my graduates have to say, visit my website at *www.RenewPT.com* and view the video testimonials. This new edition of *Ending Female Pain* is the next step in bringing my message out to a wider audience by incorporating all of my experiences into an easy-to-read woman's manual.

I've had many successes in treating women with sexual pain, and I must say that the women who are the most successful either possess or develop a positive fighting attitude and learn how to take control of their pain on their own. Taking control is not easy, but by incorporating the tools in my book you can give yourself the momentum to get the ball rolling.

When I tell people what I do for a living I often receive blank stares. Many people have either never heard of PFM dysfunction or painful sex or have never had any exposure to conditions that involve pelvic floor muscles such as interstitial cystitis, dyspareunia, vaginismus, lichen sclerosus and many more. And why would they know about these medical conditions that create havoc on women's lives? Most women enjoy sex, have no pain with penetration, have no lingering burning after orgasms, have no vulvar pain with sitting, and have no discomfort with tight clothes rubbing on their private parts. Some do not even experience any painful symptoms after childbirth. This book is written for the woman who has experienced some or all of the above symptoms, and especially for the woman who has been told things like, "There is nothing wrong" or "The pain is in your head" or "Things like that can happen."

My approach in *Ending Female Pain* is a comprehensive and empowering one. The focus is on the whole person with exercises for both mind and body. Have you ever heard the expression "It takes a village"? That's exactly how I feel about caring for women with chronic pelvic pain. Chronic pelvic pain is a complex medical condition requiring, in my opinion, a multidisciplinary medical and holistic mind-body approach. Women will have to incorporate many different treatments to help resolve their pelvic pain, and they should also know that there are other women who are experiencing the same feelings and discomforts. With this book, I hope to increase the level of dialogue and end the silent suffering of so many women out there.

If you are currently suffering from sexual pain, you will have to give up the notion that you will never get better and that this is the way things will remain. This kind of catastrophic thinking will only hinder your healing process. As you go through this book, try out all the exercises and techniques and select those that work for you. At times you may say, "These techniques don't work for me," and then you might come back a few weeks later to try them again and find that they give you great pain relief. Always keep an open mind when working with the tools in this book. Remember, every day is different. Your body will respond differently on different days.

I give my patients a lot of homework and tell them that their treatment consists of physical therapy plus independent study. You will have to put yourself first on your own list in order to heal yourself. Don't say things like, "I'm too tired tonight to do my own self-healing work." Instead, put aside all your doubts and fears, and decide to become your own savior.

I encourage you to be proactive in your own healing journey and to seek practitioners who will partner with you in your healthcare. Partnership healthcare is the only way to go. Work with caregivers who specialize in the field of pelvic pain and always follow your instincts when choosing your healthcare team. You must trust and believe in them. Select caregivers who have an open mind and are willing to try different methods, techniques, medicines and technologies to get you better. Make sure they take the time to hear what you are saying and feeling, and be sure they answer your questions no matter how trivial they may seem.

Most importantly, you must keep your head up and avoid negative self-talk. Never give up on yourself. Search for your answers with intelligence and sensibility. Always follow your own heart and intuition. If something doesn't feel right or hurts, that's an internal cue to stop and listen to your body. Do not ignore what your body is telling you.

This concept of listening to your body is especially true when you perform many of the exercises and techniques in this book. If it hurts, stop, reassess and ask yourself if this technique or exercise is the right one for you. Ask: "Am I being too aggressive with the tools? If I do this technique gently and slowly, will it hurt less and give me pain relief?" Oftentimes, the techniques you try will cause some pain as you take back control of your body, but just remember to listen to the messages your body is telling you.

Keep track of the tools and exercises that you do and become your own expert on what helps to relieve your pelvic pain. Understand that when you use the tools in this book you will have setbacks. At times, you may experience more pain. This is normal. Wait a few days and see how you feel. If symptoms flare up due to the exercises, you may feel worse for 24 to 72 hours, but eventually, you will feel better. It's the same as when you work out at the gym. There's always muscle soreness.

Now that I have covered the overall background to my mission and have primed you to get started, remember that ultimately you hold the key to your own healing. Go through this book carefully and with an open mind. You have two roads to choose from: the road to eliminate your own sexual pain or the road to stay as you are and do nothing. Read the 2nd edition of *Ending Female Pain* and make yourself the heroine of your own story.

Chapter Two

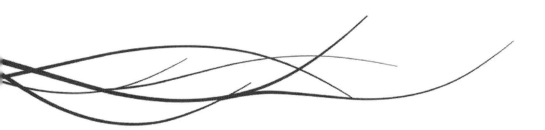

"If you are going through hell, keep going."
—Winston Churchill

Chapter 2

HOW TO USE THIS BOOK

In this book I share my trade secrets to put you on the road to a pain-free and wonderful sex life. *Ending Female Pain* represents a fusion of exercises, pain-relief techniques, and body-mind methods that I've put together to help my patients defeat their pelvic pain. Working with patients suffering from pelvic pain, I discovered a core group of exercises and techniques, that when incorporated into my patients' self-care program, helped them reduce their pain, enabled them to sit longer, allowed them to function better, and ultimately gave them back their lives. These simple-to-learn and easy-to-implement techniques helped many of my patients get rid of their sexual pain. These techniques are rolled up into "The Renew Program for Women™."

The tools are a set of holistic, natural and non-surgical methods for the treatment of female chronic pelvic pain. This unique approach incorporates several protocols that I have developed, helping many of my patients enjoy pain-free sex again or for the first time.

The large selection of techniques in this book are based on the latest medical research and on my real-life, practical experience in treating patients. The techniques include deep and superficial massage, trigger point and myofascial release, internal vaginal stretching, external pelvic muscle stretching, myofascial foam rolling, relaxation exercises, breathing techniques, and others. Above all I consider myself a coach in the lives of my patients, carefully tailoring a holistic body and mind program that works for them.

You will find that after reading this book you will become an active participant in your own self-care and treatment. You will learn how to manage and control your pain on your own, and you will feel more hopeful in your journey. *Ending Female Pain*, with its innovative methods and scientifically-based exercises, will help put you on the right track to pain-free and wonderful sex. You will be able to perform your daily chores with ease, develop a more positive outlook, and realize there are ways that you can help yourself when you experience pelvic pain flare-ups. Overall, your quality of life will improve.

What I do is physiotherapy, and what I tell my patients is that they must participate physically, emotionally, and spiritually in their treatments in order to achieve their goal of pain-free intercourse. By teaching my patients specific exercise techniques, sexual healing methods, and behavioral changes, they learn to care for themselves with the knowledge that they need to be self-sufficient and in control of their pain. At first, many of my patients feel insecure about doing the exercises and techniques on their own, but like everything else, practice makes perfect.

Exercise alone will not set you on the road to pain-free sex. You must also address your mindset and perform mental hygiene on a daily basis. Mental hygiene is extremely important. I have observed that the women I treat who are suffering from chronic pelvic pain conditions tend to be depressed. They feel hopeless because their journey has been a difficult and trying one. Many chronic pelvic pain sufferers need help with stress reduction. Many need a renewal of their spirit and soul. I believe strongly that you are what you think. Adopting a more positive outlook will help put you on the road to full recovery.

Remember that many of the women I treat have suffered pelvic pain for years. Many have gone from doctor to doctor in search of answers. Many have been told it's all in their head, or even worse, have been told to relax or to grin and bear it. Without any relief to their pain, these women are left feeling anxious, depressed and hopeless. Because of the pain that having sex brings, many avoid intimate relations with their partners resulting in strained relationships. Many endure sex even though the pain is excruciating because they fear losing their men. Other women abstain from sex and avoid being in relationships, leading to loneliness and isolation. All these emotional experiences just accumulate and add to the suffering, depression, stress and anxiety they feel. These experiences lead to catastrophic thinking and result in negative behaviors. You are not alone. I want you to use this book as a springboard to realize that there are many other women out there who are feeling the same things as you. Throughout this book I have included stories from my patients so you can see that results are out there if you work hard enough. Here is a story from one of my patients.

In Their Own Words – Finding Relief for Painful Sex

"I've had pain with sexual intercourse for years. It has been greatly affecting my relationship, my personal happiness and self-esteem. I always felt like I was the only one out there with such a problem. It was really hard for me to talk to someone about it, even close friends.

"I've seen numerous gynecologists that couldn't help me at all. Physically they didn't find anything wrong with me so they didn't know what to do with my problem. I never felt really taken cared of or listened to.

"Finally I was referred to a pelvic pain specialist that did believe in my pain being real. I thought he would be the one to finally help me. After numerous tests he diagnosed me with interstitial cystitis (IC). I was put on a very expensive medication called Elmiron® that I had to pay for out of my own pocket since I don't have proper health insurance.

"Elmiron® is a medication that really impacts your daily life because of the way you have to coordinate it with your meals. Also, you are supposed to take it for at least 3 to 6 months to see any improvement. Needless to say I wasn't happy with it, but I gave it a chance.

"It helped with urinary frequency but I did not get any relief from the pain I felt with intercourse. I felt helpless and longed to find alternatives. So I researched and spoke to people and finally ended up at Renew Physical Therapy.

"I am thrilled that I found Isa and her team. They are welcoming, understanding and comforting. They even offered a great payment plan for the physical therapy (PT) program. After an initial exam, Isa found that I had very tight muscles and started treating me and teaching me internal and external exercises to do at home.

"My doctor had never been able to find these muscular 'spasms' and tight spots. He even said specifically that PT wouldn't help me. I am proud that I took the initiative and made him prescribe PT for me regardless. You just have to really see what options you have and not just blindly listen to what your doctor tells you.

"Isa has a gift, and she knows women's bodies inside out. She has a very holistic approach to her treatment which I love. She gave me tons of tips on relaxation, nutrition, exercising, etc. But the most important part is that she empowers women to help themselves. PT is not a miracle treatment. You have to do the work yourself in order to get better. But with Isa's help and understanding, I was able to finally have sex again with much less pain than before. And I am positive that I can be completely pain free by doing my exercises."

Typical Renew Program for Women™ Routine

Ending Female Pain is best used as a foundation to your self-care and healing journey. Read the whole book before creating your first body-mind routine. By reading all four parts of the book first, you will be better able to integrate the tools and techniques into a life-changing strategy to help you take control of your pain. Remember to be gentle with yourself. If you fall off the horse, don't beat yourself up. Instead, make a decision to transform your condition and to change your outlook towards your condition from sufferer to empowered woman.

What can you expect to feel when you begin your program? You may experience emotional release, muscle soreness, or short-term exacerbation of pain. You may feel some or all of these symptoms before your momentum builds up and you begin to defeat your pain.

Your typical routine should be based on a Monday to Sunday approach. Your program needs to include activities every day of the week to combat and defeat whichever condition or combination of conditions that have led you to read this book. You will have to dedicate at least one hour per day to yourself to overcome your condition. Break up your routine into smaller parts during the course of the day, or set aside a block of time in the evening and complete your whole routine at that time. Incorporate the techniques into your daily life. Stretch at work, meditate over morning coffee, and end your day with your trigger point releases and a warm herbal bath.

Table 2.1: Typical Beginning Daily Routine

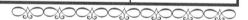

SCHEDULE	ACTION ITEM	MORE INFO
Tuesday & Thursday	Foam rolling and Pilates	Part II
Monday-Wednesday-Friday	Yoga stretching series	Part II
Daily	Hands-on self-care techniques	Part III
Daily	Kegels/reverse Kegels	Part II
Daily	Mind/Body visualizations	Part IV
Daily	Keep your mind aware of the PFM toolbox	Part IV

Mind–Body Routine

Although stress does not cause pelvic pain, it can make it worse. The stress, anxiety and emotional upheaval that accompany chronic pelvic pain can rob you of your day-to-day joys and life experiences. For best results, I recommend that you do at least one mind-body relaxation exercise every day. In times of painful flare-ups, it might be necessary to do the mind-body exercises more often and throughout the day.

I incorporate mind-body techniques into the care of my chronic pelvic pain patients as part of their strategy for success. I also encourage them to seek help from a professional who specializes in this area so they have a way to express the emotional pain they have encountered because of their conditions. The hardest thing for my patients to do is to stop the negative catastrophic thinking that accompanies pelvic pain. Many of my patients develop high levels of hyper-vigilance and "body armor" because of their sexual pain. Look to Part IV of this book for simple-to-implement and easy-to-do relaxation and mind-body techniques.

It is extremely important that all women who have chronic pelvic pain be checked out by a pelvic pain specialist to eliminate pathology and disease. It may also be necessary to seek help from a urologist or urogynecologist as many women with chronic pelvic pain also have bladder issues. Many times my patients have to augment the exercises and tools in this book with medications to ease pain, decrease spasms, elevate mood levels, control hormone levels, or deal with bladder issues. Whatever your specific medical needs are, you must have caregivers that specialize in pelvic pain as partners in your health and healing journey.

Pain Mapping/Journaling

Pain mapping is a critical component to your success. Get to know Tables 2.2 and 2.3 on pages 30 and 31 as you begin to map and rate your pain level. Table 2.2 is a basic pain-mapping chart. Use it to map your progress during your intravaginal work. For example, chart your pain like this: "My pain is in layer one at 3 o'clock rating at 8/10" (i.e., 0= no pain and 10= worst pain ever). Moving forward, you have an objective measurement to chart your progress. More details on pelvic layers can be found in Chapter 3, page 37.

Table 2.2: Mapping Your Intravaginal Pelvic Pain
PDF version of this table available at http://www.RenewPT.com

Date	Pelvic Floor Muscle Layer 1, 2, 3	Location of Trigger Point (Use the clock position)	Pain Level 0-10 (0 =no pain, 10 = worst pain)
Ex - 08-02-2009	Ex - Layer 3	Ex - 9 o'clock	7/10 pain, refers to the right labia

Recommendation: Keep a Pain and Progress Diary

Track your routine and progress in a systematic and objective manner. Doing this will let you know which techniques and exercises are working in your healing routine. Your program will evolve, but with the large selection of methods and exercises to choose from, you can mix and match until you get the perfect balance. Any worsening of your symptoms is normal in the beginning until a steady state is reached. You can download the following table at *www.RenewPT.com* so you can keep a weekly diary of your progress and pain levels.

Table 2.3: Weekly Pain and Progress Diary

PDF version of this table available at http://www.RenewPT.com

Date	Location of Pain	Pain Level 0-10 (0 =no pain, 10 = worst pain)	Techniques Used for Pain Relief	Emotional States Relaxation Technique Used
Ex - 08-02-09	Ex - Gluteal	Ex - 8/10	Ex - • Exercise • Foam Roller • Massage • Trig. Point	• Unable to relax • Soap bubbles visualization

Let's Get Started

Now that you have a road map, all you have to do is to get started. Begin today. Do not delay. Do not get overwhelmed. Sometimes it's easier to just start off slowly and then add different parts as you go. Start with things that are familiar to you. The more painful your condition, the more you will have to incorporate the techniques, methods and exercises in this book in order to manage your pelvic pain. In the beginning, you should expect to spend at least one hour a day on your "Renew Program for Women™" using the methods and exercises in this book. It is the only way to fight back. Even if you have a busy day and can only spare 5 minutes, it's better than doing nothing at all.

The self-care techniques and exercises in this book will become more familiar and easier to do the more you practice them. What I have given you are many choices. When creating your routine, choose the things that work well for you. Many of my patients become frustrated if they do not get immediate results. Be realistic. If you've had this condition for 6 months to several years, it will take time to get better. Sometimes you will feel as if you are experiencing a setback. This is quite normal as your muscles have not been worked out in this manner before. If you get really sore, cut back and be gentler with the stretches and techniques, or take a day off to rest and let your body recover. You must find the right amount of exercise for your body, your needs and your pain levels. The critical thing is not to give up but to persevere against a condition that is threatening to steal your life away from you. You must be in warrior frame-of-mind, with heart and soul strong, especially in times of painful flare-ups.

Never give up. Do something each day that brings you closer to defeating your pelvic pain. Be the heroine in your own story.

Chapter Three

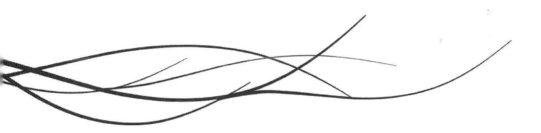

"If you're serious about changing your life, you'll find a way. If your're not, you'll find an excuse."

—Jen Sincero

Chapter 3

PELVIC FLOOR MUSCLE CONDITIONS: BACKGROUND

Before we get into the techniques, exercises and strategies for ending female pain, it is important to first understand your body on an anatomical level, a physiological level, and an energy level. Your pelvic floor is a complex set of muscles, nerves, and connective tissues like fascia that can accurately be called the cradle or basket of your being. On an energy level, the pelvic floor contains the first chakra, or energy center, and more importantly, supports the other chakras. So if the foundation is experiencing stress and trauma, then naturally all of your energy will be affected. Major nerves that innervate your entire lower extremity pass through the pelvic area, and a complex web of muscles support your vagina, bladder, uterus, intestines, and other abdominal organs. If the muscles in your pelvic floor are in spasm, or are filled with trigger points, your pain can be both excruciating and debilitating.

To understand this area of your body better, we'll take a look at the various constructs of your pelvic floor muscles, also called the levator ani muscles. We will also define conditions like vulvodynia, dyspareunia, vaginismus, and scar adhesions, and explore states of the muscle tissue like trigger points and muscle spasms. There is a lot to cover here and throughout the book, so remember to consult the extensive glossary as well to familiarize yourself with key concepts and terms found in this book.

I have also included in this chapter the basics of conducting your own visual and topical vaginal exam. You have to embrace your vagina. This may sound strange, but many of my patients are afraid to look at their vaginas which they consider ugly, or are disconnected with their pelvic floor muscles. Let me tell you straight out – your vagina is a wonderful area of your body to explore and get to know. Do not be ashamed of it. By getting to know your own anatomy and its particular nuances, you will find that you can open the door to your own healing and evolve your condition to a state of reduced pain, and more importantly, maintain long-term results. You hold the key to getting on the road to recovery.

Understanding How Your Pelvic Floor Muscles Work

Diagram 3.1: Pelvic Floor Muscles – 3rd Layer

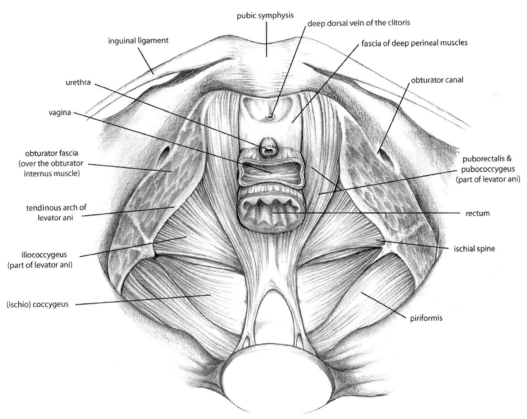

*Top down view of the pelvic floor. Your body is cut in half at the waist and you are peering down into the
3rd layer of the pelvic floor basket with organs removed. Illustration by Winston Johnson*

The overall pelvic floor muscle group has three primary functions. First, they are supportive and hold your organs up. Second, they are sphinctoric and help prevent urinary and fecal incontinence. Third, they are sexual, enhancing and making orgasms stronger and better. The pelvic

Diagram 3.2: Pelvic Floor Muscles - 1st and 2nd Layer

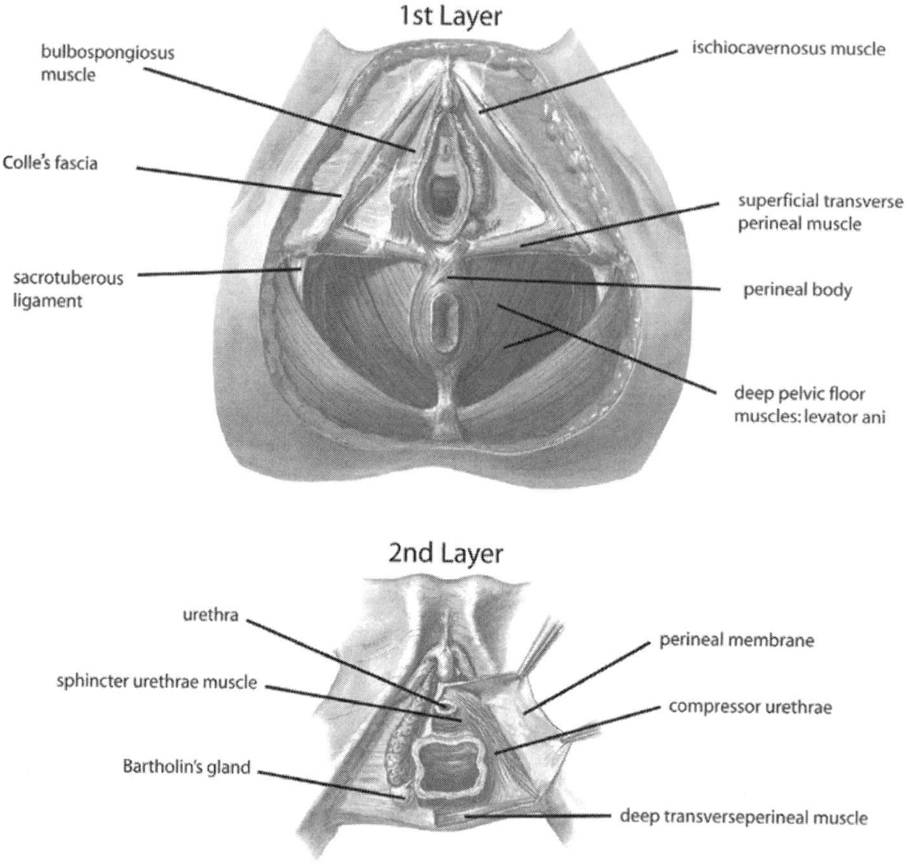

1st Layer

bulbospongiosus muscle

ischiocavernosus muscle

Colle's fascia

superficial transverse perineal muscle

perineal body

sacrotuberous ligament

deep pelvic floor muscles: levator ani

2nd Layer

urethra

perineal membrane

sphincter urethrae muscle

compressor urethrae

Bartholin's gland

deep transverseperineal muscle

The second layer muscles appear in the diagram below the first and are found behind the Layer 1 muscles listed on the top of this diagram. Source - Netter Images

floor muscles are innervated by the pudendal nerve, perineal nerve, inferior rectal nerve, the sacral spinal and levator ani nerves. These nerves originate in the low back and tailbone region anatomically known as the L4-S4 region.

The muscles of the female pelvic floor can be a source of confusion for many people – even to the trained professional – because they have been given several different names, making it difficult to understand the nomenclature and classification. In this book we will classify the female pelvic muscles into three layers and will describe other structures that are necessary to understand in order to perform the techniques described in Part III of this book. Please look at

Table 3.1 on page 38 for a description of the main muscles and anatomy of the female pelvic floor. Use the accompanying anatomy Diagrams 3.1, 3.2 and 3.3 to refer back as you begin to absorb and understand the techniques I have compiled for pelvic pain relief. Be scientific in your approach to better visualize the musculature of your own body.

The pelvic floor muscles themselves are divided into three layers, with each layer progressively deeper inside the vagina or rectum. Using your index finger as a road map, the first layer corresponds to the first knuckle, the second layer corresponds to the second knuckle and the deeper layer corresponds to the third knuckle. Now let's think about the vaginal opening looking like a clock (see Diagram 3.3). Twelve o'clock is by the clitoris, six o'clock by the rectum, three o'clock to the left side and nine o'clock to the right. Now imagine that each layer is also its own clock. So you have three clocks, one at each level,

Diagram 3.3: Pelvic Floor Muscles Layer by Layer

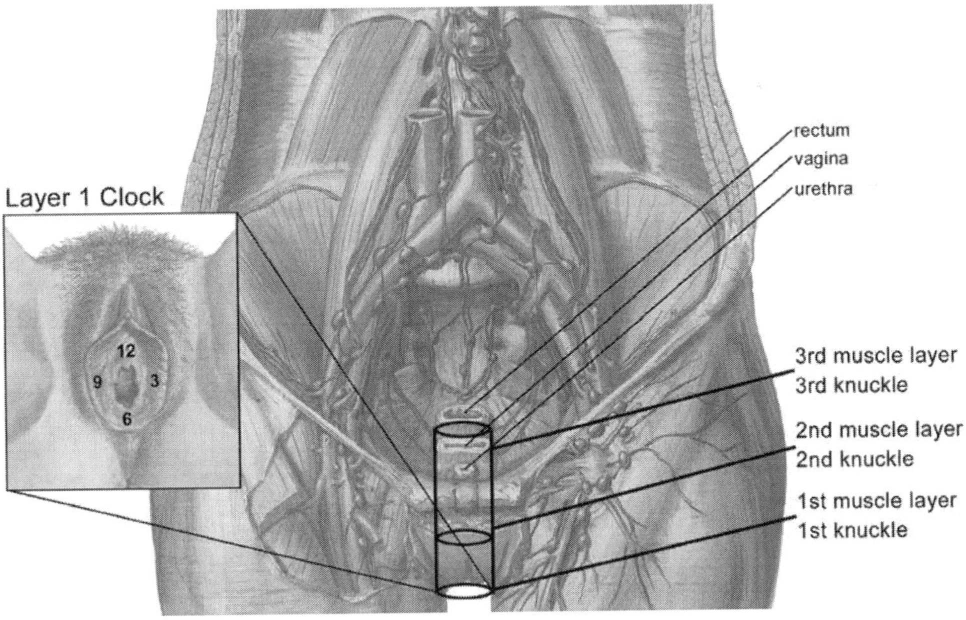

The three pelvic floor muscle layers, each corresponding to a knuckle of the index finger. The inset shows the clock concept of the 1st layer. Think of each layer as having its own clock as you begin to map and track your pain.
Source for base images: Netter Images

which is how I want you to visualize the pelvic floor muscles as you begin to digest the techniques in Part III. Thinking this way will help you locate problematic areas of your pelvic floor muscles, and will help you track your progress as you begin to understand and unravel the sources of your pain.

Table 3.1: Anatomy of Pelvic Floor Muscle Layers

LAYER NAME	MAIN MUSCLES	MAIN STRUCTURES IN LAYER
- Layer 1 - Located first knuckle of the index finger - Also called Urogenital triangle	- Superficial transverse perineal muscle - Ischiocavernosus - Bulbospongiosus - External Genitalia: includes urethra, lower vagina, vulva, mons pubis, labia majora, labia minora, clitoris, vestibular bulb, Bartholin's glands	- Colle's fascia - Vaginal/urethral openings - External female genitalia - Pubic symphysis and pubic ramibones
- Layer 2 - Located second knuckle of the index finger - Also called Urogenital diaphragm	- Sphincter urethrae - Deep transverse perineal muscle - Compressor urethrae muscle	- Bartholin's glands - Urethra - Perineal membrane - Vagina
- Layer 3 - Located third knuckle of the index finger - Also called Pelvic diaphragm	- Levator ani: Commonly broken down into pubococcygeus, puborectalis, iliococcygeus - Obturator internus - Ischicoccygeus (coccygeus)	- Tendinous arch of levator ani muscle - Obturator fascia - Sacrotuberous & sacrospinous ligament

Definitions of Muscle States –
Finding Your Trigger Points Is the First Step to Healing

Trigger points are one of the most important concepts to understand as you begin to dissect your pain. Loosely defined, trigger points are a section of muscle tissue that is stuck in its contracted state. Trigger points are knot-like spots – the most well-known example being the ones we sometimes get in our necks and trapezius muscle that create a burning and stabbing pain. Trigger points in the pelvic floor are quite similar to the ones we all get in these.

On a more anatomical and physiological level, trigger points are taut muscular bands that are the result of an injury to the motor end plate of the muscle cells. Trigger points in the pelvic floor muscles can be activated by stress, visceral or organ pain, pelvic and hip malalignment, chronic pelvic floor muscle holding, hormonal imbalances, prolonged sitting or pressure on the pelvic muscles.

Dr. Janet Travell and Dr. David Simons, pioneering experts in trigger point therapy, categorize trigger points as latent and active. The latent trigger points don't actively refer pain but cause pain when touched. Active trigger points can refer pain to another muscle or body part without actually being touched. Once trigger points are present or latent, they can become especially active with stress, strain, and injury to the muscle.

Specifically in the pelvic floor muscles, or PFMs, trigger points can elicit pain when touched or cause other symptoms like urinary urgency and frequency, feelings

Diagram 3.4: Effects of Trigger Points on Sarcomeres

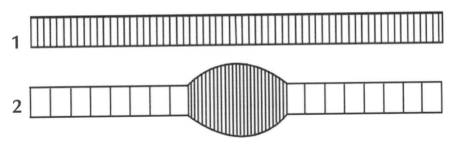

Normal muscle fibers with equidistant sarcomeres (muscle cells).
2- Trigger point shows contracted muscle fibers with outer muscle bands stretched out.

of pain with sitting, low back pain, sacroiliac (SI joint) pain, abdominal or hip pain, rectal discomfort, and pain with intercourse. Most of the trigger point techniques found in Part III will help locate and get rid of active or latent trigger points in the pelvic floor muscles, ones that when pressed cause a tremendous amount of pain or refer pain to an associated body part. Finding external trigger points that refer pain to the pelvic floor is a more difficult task, and I recommend that you work with a physical therapist that specializes in pelvic floor muscle therapy to help you make the connections to the root referral trigger point. For example, many of my patients have active trigger points in their lower backs around vertebrae L5, S1, S2 that refer pain into their pelvic floor muscles. Once located, I am able to incorporate self-healing techniques into my patients' programs, but you will need your physical therapist to do some of the detective work to unravel this part of your pain.

In conclusion, it is imperative that you begin to understand how the trigger point mechanism is at work in your own body. Once you find your trigger points, use the techniques in this book to help eliminate pain and to help reeducate the pelvic floor muscles so they have less tension, more flexibility, more range of motion, and almost always, less pain.

"The Pain Down There"

My patients want to know what caused their "pain down there." For many, their pelvic pain started acutely and then developed into a chronic condition afflicting them for months and sometimes years. Many of the women I treat tell me that their vulvar pain developed after an infection, surgical procedure, traumatic fall, or as a result of giving birth. One common thread is the devastating effects their pain has had on their lives and oftentimes on their relationships.

In my healing center, my patients report symptoms like painful sex, inability to sit for more than 10 minutes or to walk without pain, and discomfort in wearing certain clothes such as jeans, panty hose or thong underwear. Many of them suffer from sexual dysfunction or are depressed because their pain has taken their sex lives away from them. Although most of my patients are in their 20s and 30s, I also see older women suffering from these conditions as well. These women describe their pain as tingling, burning, or knife-like. Their vaginas feel raw and itchy. These symptoms can be constant or intermittent, and their pain can rate from low level to incapacitating.

Other complaints I hear from patients are clitoral pain, labial pain, groin pain, low back pain, pain in their sit bones, pain with defecation, and increased pain during their menstrual cycle. Many report vaginal dryness and redness and skin irritation that can extend to their inner thigh muscles. Others have cuts and sores in their vaginas. Some feel heaviness in their pelvis, as if there is something falling out of their vaginas. Many also describe episodes of extreme pain with penetration, called dyspareunia, and for many, this pain can linger for hours or days after their sexual encounter is over. Many tell me they have lingering pain after orgasms. One of my patients reported such intense pain after an orgasm that it made her double over in pain and cry. I have been compiling symptoms as reported by my patients for several years in an effort to discern patterns. In Table 3.2, I have created a symptoms table for you to use as a single reference to gain insight and understanding into what you are reporting as "the pain down there."

Table 3.2: Typical Symptoms of "The Pain Down There"

ORIGINS OF SYMPTOMS	SYMPTOMS AS REPORTED BY MY PATIENTS
Emotional (usually in combination with other symptoms)	- Catastrophic thinking - Isolation - Strained relationships with partners - Depression - Sadness - Guilt - Sleep disturbances - Suicidal tendencies/thoughts - Emotionally unavailable
Muscular	- Pain in the gluteal or back muscles, knees, or abdominal area - Generalized soreness in PFM muscles - PFM spasms - PFM trigger points - Constant or sharp-like pains in muscles associated or near the vagina - Pelvic floor muscle weakness
Rectal	- Bleeding with defecation - Constipation - Pain with defecation - Redness around the anus - Burning-like pain - Itching - Pushing to get feces out - Feelings of pelvic pressure - Pain in the rectum after orgasms - Pain or irritation with thong underwear
Skin	-Allergies to metals, perfumes - Sensitive skin - Irritation with certain toilet papers, tampons or sanitary napkins - Itching - Sensitivity to soaps - Painful scars - Feelings of vaginal swelling - Burning pain in the labia - Constant ache throughout the vulva - Raw feeling in the vaginal tissues

ORIGINS OF SYMPTOMS	SYMPTOMS AS REPORTED BY MY PATIENTS
Vaginal	- Painful intercourse - Vaginal itching, burning, rawness - Constant awareness of vaginal area with certain clothing - Pain with touching/wiping - Pain at opening or deep inside - Clitoral pain - Labial pain - Cuts in the vagina - Skin patches of varying colors - Pelvic pressure – feels like something is falling out of the vagina
Urinary	- Painful urination - Urgency and frequency of urination - Suprapubic pain - Hesitancy in getting urine out - Slow urine stream - Feelings of incomplete emptying - Habit of pushing urine out - Vaginal stinging with urination - Urethral pain - Feelings of pelvic pressure - Leaking with coughing, sneezing or laughing

If you have any of the symptoms I have described in Table 3.2, you might be suffering from one of the many conditions that affect the pelvic floor area. What are the most common conditions called? Most cases fall under the umbrella of vulvodynia, vestibulodynia, dyspareunia, vaginismus, interstitial cystitis, pudendal nerve entrapment, pelvic floor muscle spasm or dysfunction, lichen schlerosis, endometriosis/fibroids, and scar pain. Let's take a moment to examine each of these conditions. It is important to note that most of my patients have some combination of conditions that are contributing to their overall pain. As you take a look at each condition, you may very well discover that your symptoms point towards multiple contributing factors. Don't worry. First and foremost, we need to separate and identify each factor that is causing your pain so that you can devise the best approach to attacking and ultimately defeating the pain that is controlling your life right now.

Table 3.3: Leading Theories on the Causes of "The Pain Down There"

What Is Thought to Cause "The Pain Down There"? (Usually a Combination)
- Antibiotics
- Autoimmune disorders
- Back injuries
- Bacterial vaginosis
- Bladder problems, such as interstitial cystitis
- Candidiasis
- Childbirth causing trauma to the pelvic floor structures
- Chronic yeast infections
- Chronic infections relating to pelvic, hip muscles and abdominal organs
- Cesarean section
- Damage to nerves that innervate the pelvic area/organs or hypersensitive nerves that innervate the pelvic area
- Damage to sensory nerves of the pelvic area
- Endometriosis
- Episiotomy, perineal tearing
- Falling on coccyx or tailbone
- Fibroids
- Genital herpes
- Herniated disc
- Hip replacement surgeries and hip labral tears
- High oxalates in urine
- Hormonal problems
- Injury to the nerves that innervate the vulva
- Interstitial cystitis
- Lumbar disc problems
- Neuropathy
- Organ prolapse-bladder, uterus, or rectum
- Pelvic floor muscle spasms and trigger points
- Prolonged use of birth control pills
- Pudendal nerve damage or entrapment
- Referred pain from areas adjacent to the pelvic floor
- Repetitive stress injuries affecting the pelvis
- Sacrum injuries/surgeries

What Is Thought to Cause "The Pain Down There"? (Usually a Combination)
- Sexual abuse/rape
- Spinal fusions of the lumbar spine
- Sports injuries such as bike riding
- Straining with defecation and urination
- Surgical procedures to the pelvic/abdominal area and resulting scar adhesions
- Trauma to the pelvic area
- Trauma, injury, traction or entrapment of the pudendal nerve
- Trichomonas infections
- Vaginal atrophy secondary in menopause due to lack of estrogen
- Vulvar dermatosis

The definitive and concrete causes of all pelvic floor disorders have eluded medical professionals. What I have done here is to compile a list of the leading theories. Again, most of my patients report several causes that have contributed to their conditions.

Medical Conditions Affecting the Pelvic Floor Muscles
Vulvodynia

Vulvodynia is an umbrella term used to describe pelvic pain. There are actually several variations among which it is important to draw a distinction. Many of my patients have difficulty pinpointing their vulvar pain. They say it hurts "everywhere down there," which is called generalized vulvodynia. For others, the pain is at specific spots in their vulvas such as in their vestibules, which is called localized vulvodynia or sometimes called vestibulodynia. For some, their pain is worse during and right before their periods, or pain comes on all of a sudden, which is called unprovoked vulvodynia. Pain is sometimes also felt with direct contact to the vagina such as when wiping or with sexual intercourse. This is called provoked vulvodynia. Many also report they cannot have any penetration because the penis cannot get in the vagina (vaginismus).

The causes for vulvodynia are largely unknown and are thought to be multi-faceted. There is no evidence that vulvodynia is caused directly by sexually trans-mitted diseases or infections. Recent research has put a lot of emphasis on the nerves that innervate the pelvic and vaginal area, indicating that vulvodynia is a result of a neuropathic condition where the nerves are not functioning prop-erly. Table 3.3 lists many of the possible causes of vulvodynia. Whatever the root cause, many gynecologists, urologists and caregivers agree that the pelvic floor muscles are deeply affected, and many times normalizing their function can bring great relief to pelvic pain sufferers.

Childbirth

Childbirth is a major culprit of sexual pain and pelvic floor muscle dysfunc-tion in women. The pelvic floor muscles are stretched to their limits during delivery and the pelvic nerves also undergo traction and stretching, often com-promising their function. While these are all natural occurrences during birth, once coupled with perineal tears, episiotomies, C-sections, and assisted deliver-ies using vacuums and forceps, the birth trauma can be quickly compounded.

In obstetrics and gynecology pelvic trauma during birth is classified into degrees of tears. A first-degree tear is classified as a tear through vaginal mucosa and perineal skin only, a second degree tear is a tear that extends into the perineal muscles, a third degree tear involves a tear that extends into the external sphincter, and a fourth degree tear is a laceration affecting the anal sphincter and anal rectal mucosa. No matter what the level of the tear it is the opinion of this author that women should be routinely referred to a pelvic floor specialist after birth, and most definitely uro-gynecological rehabilitation should be prescribed routinely to all women after pelvic surgeries. In many other countries, such as France, pelvic rehab is routinely prescribed to new moms, but in the US this is not the common practice.

New moms come to me with varying complaints including pain with sitting while breastfeeding, pain with sexual intercourse, urinary leaking, fecal incontinence, perineal scar pain or C-section pain. To facilitate recovery after child-birth, I emphasize pre-natal pelvic education to solidify strategies for success. For example, pregnant women need to be empowered with information and made aware that cetain positions are less likely to cause perineal tearing.

They also need to know that perineal massage started religiously at 34 weeks of pregnancy is a great preparation for labor and helps prepare the PFMs for the upcoming stretching during labor. It is also very important for pregnant women to choose a healthcare provider who will not routinely perform episiotomies unless absolutely necessary.

Vestibulodynia

Vestibulodynia is a localized, provoked form of vulvodynia, in which particu-lar areas of the vestibule show certain characteristics. The vestibule is the oval shaped area around the opening of the vagina. This condition, sometimes also called vulvar vestibulitis is one of the most common sexual pains I treat. Vestibu-lodynia is characterized by three criteria that were first proposed by researcher Friedrich EG. Jr. in 1987, in the *Journal of Reproductive Medicine, 32:110-114.* The 3 main characteristics as described by Friedrich are:

1. Pain when the vestibule is palpated with a cotton swab. This is called the "Q-tip test" and is described in greater detail in this chapter in the section on vaginal self-examination.

2. Erythema, or redness throughout the vestibule that can sometimes extend to the labia majora and inner thighs.

3. Severe pain with vaginal penetration of the penis, speculum, tampon, finger, or dilator.

The pain felt in the vestibule is thought to be caused by a proliferation of intraepithelial nerve endings found in the vestibular mucosa. Research also shows that these nerve endings contain a compound called calcium gene related peptide. This compound is found in C-fiber nerves which are present in the vestibule. The research indicates that women with vestibulodynia have 10 times more C-fiber pain nerves in the vestibules than normal women. It is thought that this increase in C-fiber nerve endings is one of the major culprits contributing to the excruciating pain felt by women suffering from this condition.

Another possible culprit is the hyperactivity of mast cells in the vestibule. These cells play a part in the inflammatory process and also produce, among other compounds, nerve growth factor which is thought to help turn normal nerves that process pain signals into neuropathic nerves that produce pain signals no matter what the external stimulus may be.

Vaginismus

Vaginismus occurs when the muscles of the pelvic floor go into involuntary contraction, creating spasms that close the vaginal opening. Patients with vaginismus find it difficult, if not impossible, to have sex because of these severe spasms in the outer layer of the vagina. Pain in the hips, lower back, and gluteal muscles is reported as well, which makes daily activities challenging. These patients have sexual desire but the contracted muscles do not allow the penis to enter into the vagina without pain. Vaginismus is best treated with manual stretching of the pelvic floor muscles and with medical dilators as described in Part III. With proper self-care, the affected muscles release their spasms and trigger points and become softer and more supple, making sexual penetration possible.

Fibromyalgia

Fibromyalgia syndrome affects the muscles, tendons, ligaments, and soft tissues of the body. Patients generally complain of pain throughout the entire body, including the vulvar and pelvic/hip region. Additional symptoms include extreme fatigue, sleep disturbances, and burning sensations throughout the body.

Fibromyalgia sufferers have multiple trigger points and tender spots all over their bodies that when pressed elicit pain. To diagnose fibromyalgia, a good physician relies on a detailed medical history, and checks for pain and tenderness in 11 out of 18 specified trigger point areas along with locating painful areas in the body that have persisted for more than three months. For more detailed information about fibromyalgia visit a great online resource called *www.FMaware.org*.

Interstitial Cystitis

Interstitial cystitis, or IC, is a medical condition that produces pain in the bladder and urethra. IC is also known as painful bladder syndrome, and patients with IC often report symptoms of pain in the vulva, pain with intercourse, and pain in the lower back and hips. Other common complaints include urinary urgency – a feeling of an urgent need to urinate, or urinary frequency. Sometimes, the frequency can be extreme. I have had patients who go to the bathroom every 5 to10 minutes. Another common symptom is pain when the bladder is full, and patients often report that the pain subsides after urination. I recommend my IC patients keep a food diary, as there are many bladder irritants that can lead to painful flare-ups and contribute to excruciating pain if consumed. Here is a list of foods to avoid if you have been diagnosed with IC:

1. Fruit juices such as orange, cranberry, tomato, or lemon juice are bladder irritants.

2. Caffeine stimulates bladder nerves, causing pain, inflammation, and irritation to the bladder. Increased bladder nerve stimulation will also produce an increase in urinary frequency.

3. Regular or green teas because of the tannic acid found in them.

4. Regular and diet sodas because of citric acid, artificial flavoring, preserva-

tives, and carbonation.

5. Artificial sweeteners are thought to be bladder irritants.

6. Chocolate and cocoa products may irritate the bladder lining.

7. Wine and alcohol are potential bladder irritants.

For more information on IC, visit Jill Osborne's amazing web portal at *www.IC-Network.com*. She has done a great job of providing all of the latest information.

Dyspareunia

Dyspareunia is a general term that refers to painful intercourse. This pain can occur before, during, or after sexual activity. There are many causes of dyspareunia including atrophic vaginitis, vulvar vestibulitis, lichen schlerosis, endometriosis, scar adhesions, and psychological trauma such as sexual abuse.

Endometriosis

I treat many women who experience sexual pain as a result of endometriosis. The uterus is lined with a specific tissue called endometrial epithelium stroma. When this tissue grows outside of the uterus it is called endometriosis. This condition can cause a lot of pain and many other problems in a woman's body. Endometrial tissue can be found anywhere in the pelvis, such as the ovaries, uterus, fallopian tubes, intestines, bladder and colon. Most women with endometriosis usually experience pelvic pains during their menstrual cycles, but many also have excruciating pain that is not related to their periods. Endometriosis can cause not only sexual pain but also infertility, as the tissue growths can affect fallopian tubes, ovaries and the proper functioning of the uterus.

If adhesions and scar tissue related to endometriosis build up, it can lead to a condition called frozen pelvis. If you think you are suffering from endometriosis you must make sure you are comfortable with your caregivers. Find one who always works closely with a gynecologist that specializes in endometriosis, as surgery is often performed in conjunction with physical therapy to achieve results.

Adhesions/Scar Pain

Post-surgical scar adhesions occur in women after most pelvic and abdominal surgeries. An adhesion is a fibrous band of scar tissue that forms between internal organs and tissues, joining them together abnormally. Adhesions form after surgery as part of the normal healing process and help to limit the spread of infection. Sometimes though, adhesions cause tissues to grow together that normally would not be connected. Millions of people worldwide suffer from painful adhesions after surgery, and data has suggested over 50 percent of women will develop scar adhesions following gynecologic and non-gynecological surgeries (Obmanagement.com, June 2003, Vol. 15, No. 6). In my experience, the longer a woman waits to seek therapy for her scars, the denser and tougher the scar adhesions become. More importantly, scar adhesions may be associated with pelvic pain and sexual pain, abnormalities of bowel function, and infertility.

I have seen many women develop overall pelvic pain because of adhesions after surgical procedures such as C-sections, myomectomy, hysterectomy, laparoscopic procedures, episiotomy, vestibulectomy, hymenectomy, perineal tearing, and even vulvar biopsies.

How to Perform a Self-Examination of the Vulva-Vaginal Area

Now that you have a basic understanding of the symptoms, general causes and various conditions that can afflict pelvic floor muscles and tissues, it is important to take the time to get to know your own body. You cannot be successful with your own self-care unless you take the time to examine yourself and learn to understand the uniqueness of your body. Many of the women I treat start out in my healing center completely disconnected to their pelvic floor muscles and vaginas. I tell them that they have to change this outlook in order to have any chance of success. Get to know your body first so you can get on the road to recovery and long-term results.

Make sure to perform your exam in a well-lit place. If the area you are in is poorly lit, you will need additional lighting. You will also need a mirror, Q-tip and lubricant.

There are many positions in which you can perform your vulva examination. It is important to find a position that you are comfortable in and allows you to examine the whole area. Recommended positions for this examination are sitting with legs apart or standing with one leg up or squatting over a mirror.

Hold your mirror up close to examine all the external parts. To examine the inner parts you will have to spread your vaginal lips to expose the vulvar area.

Checking All the Parts

The vulva is made up of the following structures: labia majora, labia minora, clitoris, vestibule of the vagina, bulb of the vestibule, and the glands of Bartholin. We will also be examining the perineum in addition to the vulva.

Diagram 3.5: External Genitalia, Part of Layer 1 of the Pelvic Floor Muscles

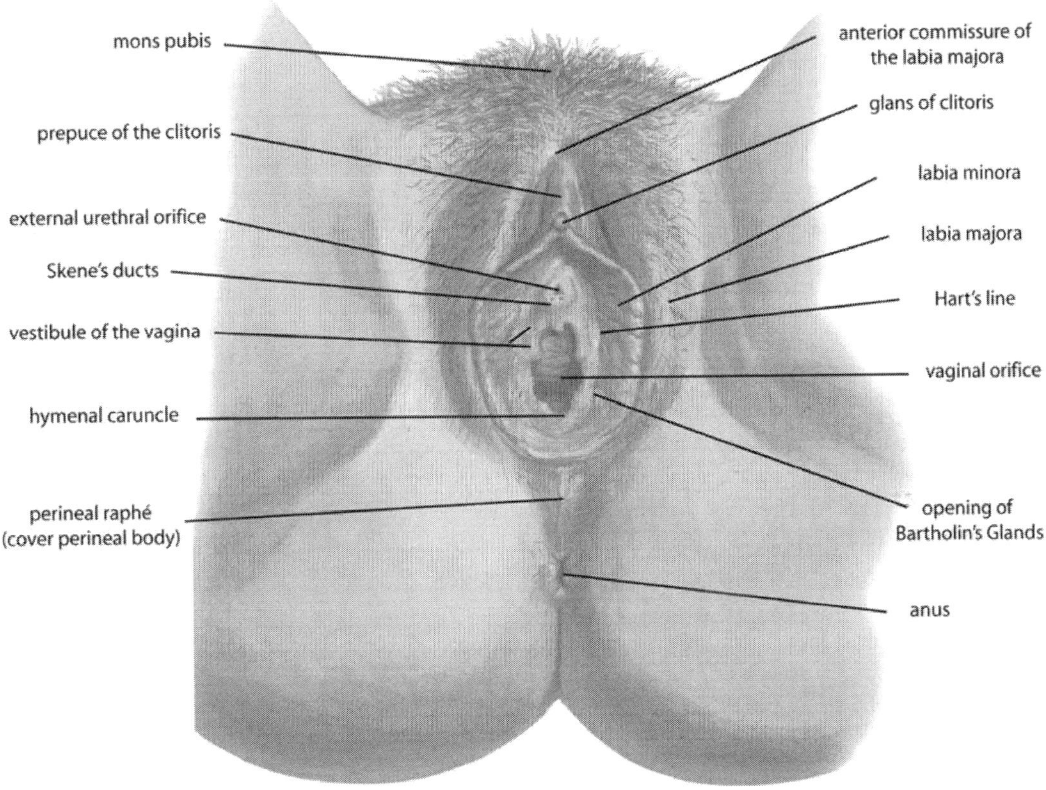

mons pubis

prepuce of the clitoris

external urethral orifice

Skene's ducts

vestibule of the vagina

hymenal caruncle

perineal raphé
(cover perineal body)

anterior commissure of
the labia majora

glans of clitoris

labia minora

labia majora

Hart's line

vaginal orifice

opening of
Bartholin's Glands

anus

Base image: Netter Images

Check Your Mons Pubis

This is the area where your pubic hair and pubic bone are located. Some-times this is an area of pain for some women who have bladder conditions.

What to Look For

Run your fingers along the skin and feel for any bumps, warts, or sores. Also examine the area for any color changes in the skin such as red, white or dark spots.

Check Your Clitoris

Feel and look at your clitoris and the surrounding area. Also gently pull back on the hood of the clitoris.

What to Look For

Does the clitoral hood move or is it bound down? The clitoris should freely move in its hood. Also examine the clitoris for coloring, pain and inflammation by lightly touching over it with your finger or Q-tip.

Check Your Labia Minora

These are the inner lips to the right and left of the vaginal opening.

What to Look For

Look and touch by holding the labial skin between thumb and fingers. Check on all sides of the labias – front and back and both sides right and left. Run your fingers along the skin and feel for any bumps, warts, or sores. Examine the area for any color changes in the skin such as red, white or dark spots. Look for ulcers, sores, small blisters, and areas of pain, swelling and inflammation. This area can appear very red and inflamed in women with pelvic floor dysfunction and in women suffering from vulvar vestibulitis.

Check Your Labia Majora

These are your outer vaginal lips next to the labia minora. Slide your fingers along the outer lips both sides. Many of my patients have labial pain, trigger points or itching along the length of the outer labias. Massage and cross friction massage, covered in Part III, work great in reducing pain in this area.

What to Look For

Perform the same examination as for the labia minora.

Check Your Perineum

Although the perineum and the vestibule, the area that surrounds your vaginal opening, are typically not included in the vulva self-examination, I highly recommend that you do not overlook them in your monthly self-care examination. Examining these areas will give you tremendous insight into your pelvic pain condition.

The perineum is the area between your vagina and anus. This is where doctors perform an episiotomy, which is a surgical cut of the perineum done just before the delivery of a child. Many women who experience pain have scar tissue in this area as a result of the episiotomy. This area is a highway for many muscles and it provides us with an external view of the levator ani muscles, also known as pelvic floor muscles. Palpation or touching of this area will give you an idea about what is going on internally in your pelvic floor muscles such as mobility and pain.

What to Look For

First, look for scar tissue, lesions, and sores. Also examine the area for any color changes in the skin such as red, white or dark spots. Many times this area becomes red and hyper-irritable due to the dysfunction that is present in the pelvic floor muscles. When the muscles of the vagina function better, the redness and irritation in this area disappears. You will need a mirror and to be in a well-lit room for this exam as well.

Now look at the perineal body. This is the midpoint of the perineum. Testing this area for mobility and ease of movement will give you an insight to what is going on in your pelvic muscles. When performing your pelvic drops, pelvic floor muscle release, or reverse Kegels, this is the area you want to see drop down, release or come forward towards your mirror. Many times I will instruct my patients to gently move this area to the left, right, up, and down and to feel which direction it is not moving freely. Once you have established that, stretch the perineal body into that direction by holding it in the stretch position for 30 seconds to one minute. I cover this in greater detail in Part III.

Q-tip Test

The Q-tip test is an essential method for determining the levels of inflammation and pain in the vestibule. As you progress on your healing journey, you will continually perform the Q-tip test and track your results. In ideal settings the Q-tip test should elicit no pain. If you experience any pain with this test, consult a physician or physical therapist that specializes in pelvic pain immediately.

Where is the vestibule? The vulvar vestibule forms an oval shape around the opening of the vagina. The top is bordered by the clitoris, the bottom by the posterior fourchette, the inner sides by the hymenal remnants and the outer parts of the oval by the labia minora. Additional structures found in the vulvar vestibule include the major and minor vestibular glands, Skene's Gland and the urethra.

Diagram 3.6: Location of Hart's Line

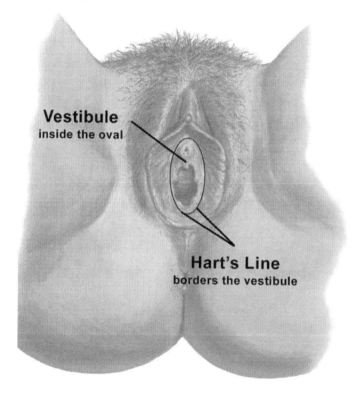

Perform the Q-tip test along Hart's Line
Base images: Netter Images

To perform this test you will need a mirror and a Q-tip with a small amount of lubricant. Locate the line that separates the labia minora from the vestibule. This is called Hart's Line. Once you locate it with your mirror, imagine the vestibule as a clock, with the clitoris at twelve o'clock, the left at three o'clock, the anus at six o'clock, and the right at nine o'clock. Using very gentle pressure, go around the clock from one o'clock to twelve o'clock. As you perform this test, rate the level of pain you experience from 0 to 10 (i.e., 0 = no pain, 5 = moderate pain, 10 = worst pain ever). If this test elicits any pain you probably have some form of vestibulodynia. Make sure to keep track of your painful areas with your Q-tip.

Vaginal Scars

During your examination, you may come across old scars that you may not have noticed before. Scars and tears in the perineum can often be a source of sexual pain. Vaginal scars are frequently the result of episiotomies or tearing during childbirth, or surgical procedures such as biopsies and vestibulodectomies. It is possible for the perineum to tear during childbirth or sexual activity. Check out your scars for proper healing, pain and mobility. If the scar feels thick, is painful or has a discharge, have it checked by your gynecologist. If the scar is raised, painful, thick or feels tight, there are ways to reduce pain, stretch the scar, and restore motion to the tissues. Trigger points may exist in these perineal scars and refer pain to the vulva and pelvic floor muscles. See Part III of this book for treatment and healing techniques for perineum scars.

Diagram 3.7: Clock Concept for Hart's Line Test

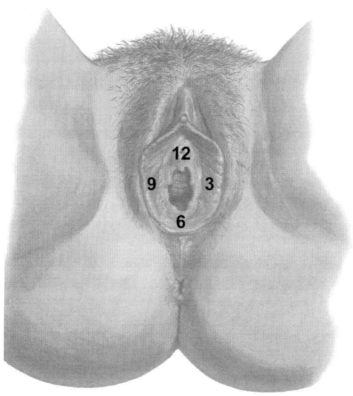

Base image: Netter Images

We've just covered the basics of your pelvic floor muscles and structures, both internally and externally. Remember you must get to know your own anatomy, with its nuances and uniqueness. Now let's get ready in this next section of the book where we will build our foundation, with Kegels, ball strengthening, yoga stretching, at-work strategies, and foam rolling.

Part 2
Exercises and Stretches for the Relief of Pelvic Pain

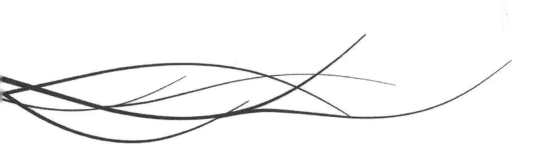

"We are what we repeatedly do.
Excellence, therefore,
is not an act but a habit."
— Aristotle

Chapter 4

TO KEGEL OR NOT TO KEGEL

The term *Kegel*, developed by gynecologist Dr. Arnold Kegel, is used to describe a set of exercises that is designed to improve the function of the pelvic floor muscles. The problem is that there are subtle nuances to Kegels that if not taken into account, can actually produce worse results for patients with pelvic pain. Typically, basic Kegels are prescribed for women suffering from incontinence or organ prolapse, and are designed to help strengthen the PFMs, improve coordination, continence and sexual function by reducing laxity and decreasing weakness.

When I evaluate a typical woman suffering from pelvic pain, I frequently find that in addition to muscle weakness, the PFMs usually have excessive tone, increased shortness, extreme tension, spasms and multiple trigger points in them, rather than laxity. I also often find a lack of flexibility in the muscles that attach to the pelvis such as the inner thighs, hip flexors, gluteal and abdominal muscles. The PFMs are normally in a relaxed state, and they respond to what is happening in your body and mind. They can respond to thoughts, past experiences, trauma, visceral problems, abnormal breathing patterns and pain. Usually, their response to any of the above is to become tense. This tension can go on for years, resulting in shortened muscle fibers filled with spasms, trigger points, and myofascial restrictions.

Once the muscle fibers get shorter and tenser, they are typically weaker. The weakness is not due to looseness, as in the typical incontinence or prolapse patient. Instead, the weakness is caused by muscles which are too tight or hypertonic. The shortened muscle has the ability to contract, but the contractions are weak because there is a decrease in the fiber's ability to move. This type of weakness leads to urinary leaking and urge and frequency of urination, which are typical complaints I hear from my patients with pelvic pain. To effectively treat these hypertonic muscle fibers, they first need to be lengthened and relaxed before they can be strengthened and toned. So the prescription of regular Kegels, where you are told simply to draw up your muscles to prevent leaking or pain, does not work. In fact it can lead to more pain and weakness as muscle fibers become even shorter, and more hypertonic. As a result, the PFMs often develop more trigger points in them.

In order to accomplish the release, I recommend that my patients do a daily, reverse Kegel release program first and then embark on a Kegel strengthening program for their muscles once they master the muscle relaxation and release techniques. Having first lengthened the muscles, the fibers can then be better strengthened, leading to reduced pain, improved continence, and enhanced sexual response.

The Kegel programs I have created are to be performed on several levels, beginning with the reverse Kegels to relax the muscles, followed by strengthening with the contract, relax, and the quick-flicks Kegels once you have mastered the reverse series. This order is necessary because the release is needed first before you can strengthen both slow twitch and fast twitch fibers of the PFMs. By understanding some of the nuances of the types of Kegels. I will describe in the following paragraphs, you can achieve better success and gain better control over your pain.

Reverse Kegel Muscle Relaxation Series

Your ability to have conscious release of the pelvic floor muscles is a critical part of your recovery program. The foundation of conscious and mindful release is the mastering of the reverse Kegel relaxation exercises. Your success in all of the other techniques in Part III of this book rests on the reverse Kegel series I describe in this chapter. You must learn to focus on and relax these muscles before they·can become functional again and pain-free. Relaxation and lengthening of the PFMs with reverse Kegels is also called downtraining. To ensure success with your overall program, you need to do reverse Kegels and downtraining along with the techniques in Part III of this book, which include PFM massage, trigger point, pressure, and myofascial release as well as intravaginal dilator stretching.

The reverse Kegel downtraining series contains eight techniques that will help you gain awareness and control over your pelvic floor. In the beginning, work hard to master the release techniques, and then you can incorporate this focus while performing the other sexual healing tools throughout this book. It is extremely important that you practice your relaxation exercises throughout the day. Do not go through an 8-hour work day without releasing the tension in your muscles. The following exercises are easy to perform and can be done anywhere or anytime. At first the PFM relaxation exercises will be extremely difficult to visualize and perform. Many of you have had tension and pain in these muscles for a very long time. Like anything else, the more you practice these exercises, the easier they will become to do and to implement. The reverse Kegel series in this book contains the most effective methods that have brought success to my patients. Designed to help you release the tension and then strengthen the PFMs, they are to be used on a daily basis, and especially during flare-ups when they could be used every hour until the pain subsides.

The Importance of Breath

To more effectively perform the reverse Kegel series, you must couple the techniques with proper breathing. When I teach my patients the basics of downtraining, I emphasize diaphragmatic breathing to ensure their success. Diaphragmatic breathing can be defined as a type of breathing that involves the abdominal muscles instead of the ribs, shoulders, and neck muscles. To practice diaphragmatic breathing, place your hand over your belly button. On inhale, let your belly gently rise out into your hands, and on exhale, let the belly flatten. Don't let the breath raise your shoulders, and don't bring your belly in on the inhale and out on the exhale, as this is not diaphragmatic breathing.

The best way to consciously release tension from the PFMs is to try to release the muscles while you inhale. Do not be discouraged if you find this difficult to perform. All of my patients have trouble with this concept in the beginning. Just imagine though, that when you inhale properly, your diaphragm actually lowers to make room for the air, so it is natural to also lower and relax the pelvic floor muscles. When you exhale, your diaphragm rises to push the air out, and you can then raise or contract your PFMs.

It is also important to time your inhalation and exhalation so that they occur over the same length of time. For example, inhale for five seconds, and then exhale for five seconds. I usually recommend to my patients that they inhale for a count of five while consciously dropping and relaxing their PFMs downward. This release and letting go is the hardest exercise to do because many women are not even aware of the tension with which they are holding their PFMs. Once the tension is released, the muscle fibers begin to lengthen. Soon you will be able to release on demand, at which point you can begin a regular Kegel strengthening and toning program.

If you have difficulty coordinating the in-breath with the release, don't let that stop you. It's perfectly alright to do a reverse Kegel with exhalation at first until you master the correct techniques. The most important thing is to increase your awareness and focus and to practice reverse Kegels on a daily basis, even an hourly basis, if needed.

Test Your Progress

Table 4.1: The Renew Physical Therapy Reverse Kegel Self-Grading System

PROGRESS LEVEL	CURRENT CONDITION	ACTION TO BE TAKEN
Level 1	Not able to release PFM	Continue with PFM Release Exercises
Level 2	Able to release PFM a little	Continue with PFM Release Exercises
Level 3	Able to release PFM but not all the way and with some pain	Continue with PFM Release Exercises
Level 4	Able to release PFM completely without pain or with some pain	Start Kegel Strengthening Contract/Relax Program

You should continue practicing your reverse Kegel program until you feel like you are gaining control over your muscles. The only way to tell if you have complete relaxation is to test your PFM by inserting a finger into your vagina and grading the release. I have created a 4-level grading system and included it in Table 4.1 so you can accurately evaluate your progress. This is the most accurate way to test because I find many of my patients think they are releasing when in reality they are contracting the muscles and creating more pain. When you test yourself, grade yourself on a scale of 1-4. A grade of 3 or 4 should be achieved before starting your Kegel strengthening contract/relax program.

What will you feel with your finger during your reverse Kegel self-grade test? You should feel the tension or grip around your finger releasing, and the finger should gently slip outward. You can also use a mirror to better visualize the reverse Kegel. When using a mirror, you should see the muscles come towards the mirror. You should also see the perineal body, or area between the vagina and the rectum, drop down towards the mirror. If you see this area lifting up, you are doing the reverse Kegel series incorrectly. Also look at your anus with the mirror. The anus should open up as if you were passing gas, but not pushing out, which is a sign of bearing down and straining. Again, if you see the anus contract and pull in, you are performing the reverse Kegel incorrectly.

Table 4.2: Reverse Kegel Downtraining Series

TECHNIQUE
1. Rose Petal Flower Release
2. Direct Vaginal Release
3. Child's Pose Release
4. Prayer Squat Release
5. Dead Bug Release
6. Mini-Squat Release
7. Side Lying Sit Bones Apart Release
8. Dropping the Panties
9. Body Check Release

Reverse Kegel Downtraining Series

Rose Petal Flower Release

WHAT TO DO:

As you breathe in for 5 to 7 seconds, send your inhalation breath to your vaginal muscles visualizing and imagining them as a large tight rose flower that is beginning to blossom in the springtime. Imagine the rose opening up petal by petal. Try this exercise for 5 breaths.

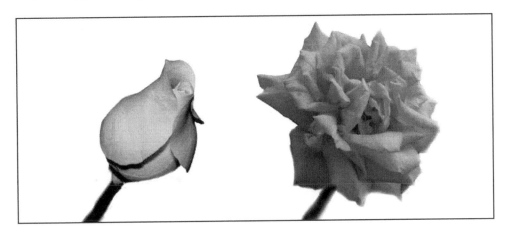

Direct Vaginal Release

WHAT TO DO:

1. Place your clean, gloved finger or dilator into your vagina. Try to find a position that is comfortable for you to maintain your finger in your vagina for at least 5 minutes. You can try different positions such as standing, sitting or lying on your side and find the one that works best for you. At times you may be able to do a PFM release in one position but not another. It is important to try all positions to enhance PFM relaxation in any position.

2. As you breathe in, send your in-breath into your vagina and imagine that the walls of your vagina are expanding away from the dilator or finger. If you are using a dilator, you should feel the dilator gently and slowly slip out of the vagina as you do your relaxation exercises.

3. If your dilator/finger is being pushed out as you do your direct release then you are forcing the release and putting undue stress and strain on your pelvic muscles. Pushing to get the release is not the same as gently allowing it to happen with your in-breath. Always couple the visualization with the inhalation.

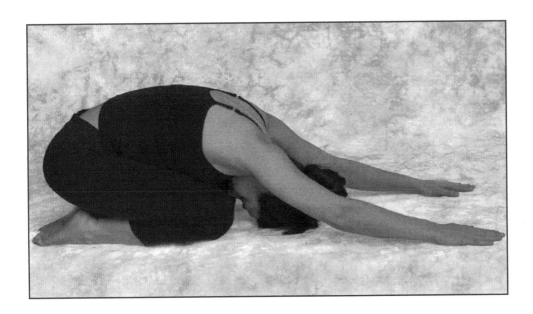

Child's Pose Release

WHAT TO DO:

1. Go on your hands and knees and then bring your body into child's pose as in the above photo. Bring one hand onto each sit bone and keep contact with the bones as you perform your PFM relaxation child's pose release.

2. If your sit bones do not touch your heels, place a pillow under your gluteal muscles and feet. Now imagine as you breathe in for a count of 5 seconds that your sit bones are moving away from each other. Simultaneously feel your pelvic muscles release and relax. Make sure your in-breath lasts as long as the pelvic release (at least 5 seconds), and then perform for 5 breaths.

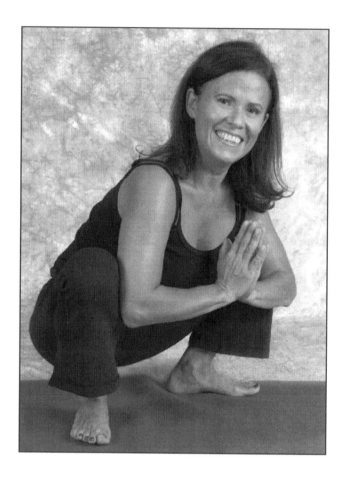

Prayer Squat Release

WHAT TO DO:

1. Get into the Prayer Squat Position as photographed in the above photo. It's best to hold on to a sturdy object when performing this exercise to facilitate the pelvic floor muscle release and to reduce any undue stress this exercise can put on the thighs, back and calf muscles.

2. If your heels do not touch the floor, place a pillow under your heels to make this exercise more comfortable and less stressful.

3. Send your in-breath into your vaginal pelvic floor muscles for a count of 5 seconds.

4. You can remain in this position for 10 releases or you can get up and down within each repetition.

5. Aim to be in this position for 5 minutes a day.

6. While performing the exercises, focus on inhalation breathing, making sure not to hold your breath.

Dead Bug Release

WHAT TO DO:

1. Lie on your back, bring your knees to your chest and place one hand on the inside of each knee.

2. While inhaling, imagine your sit bones coming apart and your pelvic muscles releasing. Inhale for at least 5 seconds, exhale and repeat for 5 breaths.

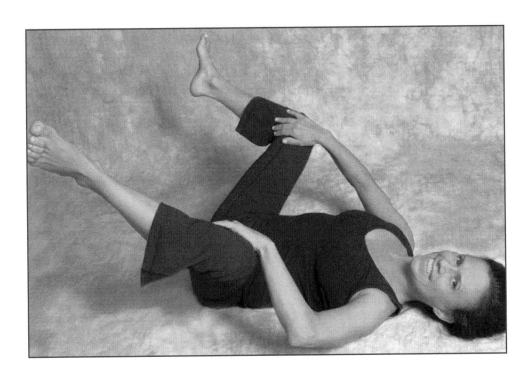

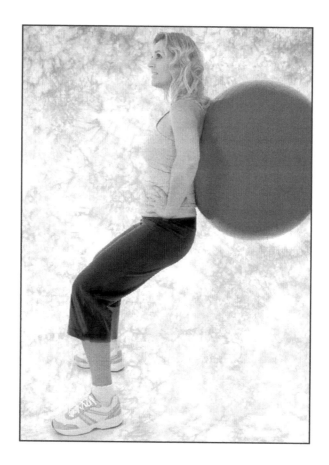

Mini-Squat Release

WHAT TO DO:

1. While standing with feet hip-width apart, knees slightly bent and in good postural alignment, place one hand on each hip bone. You can use a ball as in the photograph if it is too difficult

2. Imagine you are about to sit in a chair and perform a mini-squat, while focusing on inhaling into your PFM and simultaneously visualizing your sit bones coming apart. Lower your body for 5 seconds as you breathe in and go back to start position as you exhale.

3. Repeat 10 times or do as many as you can tolerate. This exercise is great because it works with gravity to get you the PFM release and at the same time strengthens your legs.

Side Lying Sit Bones Apart Release

WHAT TO DO:

1. Lie down on your right side and place your left hand on your left sit bone.

2. As you breathe in, pull the left sit bone away from the right. Feel and imagine your pelvic floor muscles dropping outward, relaxing and releasing.

3. Hold this release for 5 seconds, go back to neutral or start position and repeat for 5 breaths.

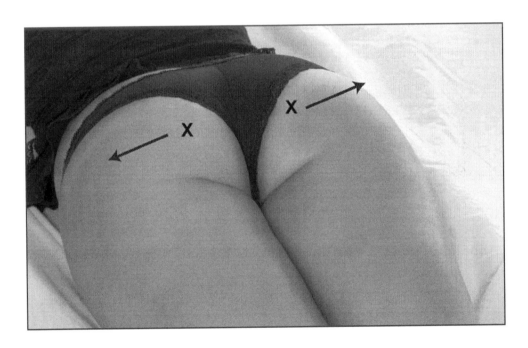

The X's represent the location of the sit bones' release. The arrows represent the way you should imagine your sit bones moving while you are in side lying position.

Dropping the Panties

WHAT TO DO:

1. Sit with good posture with your weight evenly distributed on your sit bones.

2. Practice diaphragmatic breathing for several minutes to center yourself.

3. Breathe in for a count of 5 and imagine that your panties and vaginal muscles are dropping into the chair.

4. Make sure to direct your in-breath to your PFM. With your visualization, collect your pelvic pain and imagine the pain leaving your body with your exhalation or out-breath.

Body Check Release

WHAT TO DO:

1. In any position, start with 1 to 2 minutes of diaphragmatic breathing to center yourself .

2. Tune into your muscles, and ask yourself, "Where are my muscles in space and in what state are they in?"

3. Practice releasing the muscles with the inhalation breath.

4. This technique should be utilized during stressful times such as when you are arguing with someone, and also during periods with painful flare-ups.

Traditional Kegel Contract/Relax Series

Congratulations! If you are reading this section and getting ready to move into the contract/relax series, then you are doing really well with the downtraining! Take a conscious moment to congratulate yourself for getting this far. For women in this phase of their recovery, I like to start them with a contract/relax program.

Start by examining your PFMs. Perform an internal vaginal examination with your index finger, similar to the self-grading exam for the reverse Kegels. During this self-exam you need to find out how many seconds you can hold a contraction and conversely how many seconds it takes you to release your muscles completely. These 2 numbers will determine a ratio that you will use as a starting point of your contract/relax program.

How to Determine Your Contract/Relax Program Ratio

1. Please have a mirror and lubrication on hand for your exam.

2. Start off by first looking externally at your perineum and performing a contract Kegel.

3. For correct Kegel execution look for the following motions: your clitoris should move slightly downward, your anus should wink, and the perineal body should move up and in.

4. After looking at your Kegel contraction, look at your reverse Kegel. You should see the anus release and your perineal body move outwards towards the mirror.

5. Once you are performing the Kegel and the reverse Kegel correctly, place a well-lubricated index finger into your vagina and contract your PFM around your finger. Count to see how many seconds you can hold the contraction by counting 1 Mississippi, 2 Mississippi, 3 Mississippi, etc. Stop counting once you feel the contraction of the Kegel get weaker or release. This is the number of seconds to use for the contract.

6. Start releasing your muscles and see how many counts of Mississippi it takes you to release your PFM completely. From these 2 numbers, determine your contract/relax ratio. For example, you might start out with a 5-second Kegel contraction and a 10-second release so your ratio would be 1:2.

7. Always err on the side of safety by giving yourself more time to release.

Kegel Strengthening Program

Contract/Relax and Slow/Relax

1. Now that you have determined your ratio, start your strengthening program conservatively by performing 10 repetitions of contract/relax 3 times daily, incorporating your ratio as your guide.

2. Pay close attention to make sure your pelvic pain does not increase with your current strengthening program. If you start to experience more pain, stop the contract/relax exercises immediately and go back to the relaxation exercises and/or the internal work described in Part III.

3. After 1 to 2 weeks, if you are doing well with your contract/relax program, start doing your program 4 to 5 times daily.

4. After 2 weeks, retest to see if your PFM contract endurance has improved. If it is longer, then add more seconds to your contraction Kegel. For example, after 2 weeks of diligently doing your strengthening exercises, you can now hold your slow Kegels for 7 seconds. Then start doing your program with 7 seconds contract and 14 seconds release, using the same 1:2 ratio as a guide. You may find your ratio changes over time, and if so, this is acceptable.

Quick-Flick Kegels

In conjunction with your contract/relax Kegel, add the quick-flick Kegel exercises as well. These consist of 1 to 2 second contracts followed by 1 to 2 second releases, repeated 10 to 20 times. These quick Kegels should be performed after resting for 1 minute after the slow Kegels.

For strengthening programs, the goal that I usually set for my patients is a 10-second slow Kegel contraction with a 10 to 20 second release, performed 3 to 5 times daily. After one set of the slow Kegels, I recommend waiting 1 minute and then doing 10 to 20 quick Kegels. By performing both types of Kegel strengthening exercises, you will hit the slow twitch and fast twitch muscle fibers of the pelvic floor.

Correct Kegel downtraining followed by Kegel strengthening is part of the foundation of your healing journey. As you master your Kegel program in conjunction with the self-massage and intravaginal techniques found in Part III of this book, you will be armed with some very powerful tools that can help you regain a pain-free life. Do not quit if you find yourself feeling frustrated with your breathing and releasing on the inhale. Be content to make small improvements if needed, in the beginning. You will achieve breakthroughs as long as you continue to persevere.

Strive for a deep understanding of your body so that you can remain aware of your PFMs with your day to day activities.

In the next chapters, you will be doing contract/relax Kegels while performing physio ball strengthening, and you will also do reverse Kegels while releasing stress at work and with your yoga program.

In Their Own Words – One Woman's Search for Answers

"My pain started 8 years ago when I had sex with a new partner. It was a pain I was unfamiliar with – burning and abrasive. My first thought was that I had a yeast infection so I consulted a nurse-midwife. She confirmed the presence of yeast and prescribed boric acid capsules especially formulated by a compounding pharmacy. I tried this as well as garlic cloves inserted as pessaries, off and on for a year or so. The pain would come and go; at times increasing dramatically with normal activities like sitting and walking to the subway. These times, I felt the pain more intensely as if being stabbed or burned.

"Realizing this was not a yeast infection, I went back to the nurse-midwife. She told me later that she suspected I had vulvodynia, but didn't want to diagnose me herself. She sent me to a respected OB/GYN in a large practice. The doctor confirmed her suspicion; but when I asked about treatment options, I was horrified. They included using novocaine to numb the area; applying estrogen cream; taking antiseizure and antidepressant drugs like Neurontin; and finally, surgery to remove the painful areas. In the meantime, the doctor recommended I have a glass of wine and try to relax the next time I had sex.

"I did not find comfort until some time later when a new OB/GYN recommended physical therapy; specifically, internal trigger point and myofascial release. She referred me to Isa's practice where I have been going for a few months now. Since starting the therapy, I see a huge improvement. Isa told me that having a dysfunctional pelvic floor for years has caused other body parts to be affected. By this time, I was also experiencing pain in my hip joints and lower back.

"So far, the result has been wonderful! Not only am I experiencing less pain, I am also learning a lot about the interconnections of the pelvis, hips and back muscles, and how to keep them all talking to each other happily through manual release of trigger points, the use of a foam roller, and stretching. I don't mind that the program has required a lot of work from me because the results are immense. It is such a relief to know there is a valid treatment for this pain. It is not just psychological, and now I have a whole arsenal of tools to stay in control of my pain."

Chapter Five

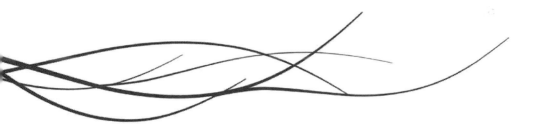

"Optimism is the faith that leads to achievement. Nothing can be done without hope or confidence."

— Helen Keller

Chapter 5

THE HERRERA PILATES BALL STRENGTHENING ROUTINE FOR PELVIC PAIN™

Overcoming your pain and getting on the right track to long-term management of your condition requires a multidisciplined approach. One of the important disciplines you will have to undertake is to get yourself on a basic strengthening program to better align and hold your body. I have developed a great workout for my patients which I will share with you in this chapter. Based on Pilates and using the physio ball, this concentrated and focused routine targets areas that are often weakened and shut down by pelvic pain.

In the beginning, do all of the exercises in the routine. As you gain confidence and strength, mix and match to come up with your own sets and routines that give you the most targeted relief. Remember to listen to your body while doing the Pilates ball exercises. Don't overdo it too soon, especially if you are not someone who has worked out much before reading this book.

Many of the lower extremity muscles in women with pelvic pain become shortened, tight and weak. Upper body muscles also become weak, contributing to poor postural alignment and pain. To regain balance in your body you must focus on a toning and strengthening program as one of the foundational blocks from which you can achieve and maintain long-term results. An overall program that incorporates upper and lower body strengthening will balance out the weaknesses, promote a healthier body, and propel you forward with the other disciplines and techniques highlighted throughout this book.

From my experience, women who suffer from pelvic pain usually have comparable body-types and similar muscular weaknesses. It is the nature of this condition for the body to often draw inwards, creating postural issues like forward head, rounded shoulders, slouching into the lower back, and general weakness in the hips. Everything in the body is connected either directly or indirectly, so it is very important to include an overall strengthening program as one of the building blocks to your long-term recovery.

How to Purchase a Physio Ball

You will need to purchase a physio ball for the strengthening and yoga series. The balls usually come in four different sizes depending on the height of the user. Use Table 5.1 as a reference when you purchase your physio ball. In addition to doing the yoga series with the ball, I love to do basic stretches and strengthening, as well as pelvic floor muscle exercises, as it helps break the boredom. It is a great tool that will help support you if you find that a stretch or exercise is too difficult, and you will find that using the ball challenges your stabilizing muscles in unique ways.

Table 5.1: Physio Ball Height Guidelines

Height of User in Feet & Inches	Size of Ball in Centimeters
4' 7" – 5' 0"	45 cm ball
5' 1" – 5' 6"	55 cm ball
5' 7" – 6' 1"	65 cm ball
6' 2" – 6' 8"	75 cm ball

Specific Considerations for Your Pelvic Floor Muscles When Performing the Pilates Series

1. Very important! If you are still downtraining your PFMs and have not reached the contract/relax phase of your Kegel program, you can still perform the Pilates ball series to create balance and strength. If this is the case, keep your abdominals pulled in at 30% effort and fo-

cus on keeping your PFMs relaxed throughout the entire exercise series. If you are performing your contract/relax Kegels, then choose only 3 of the 10 exercises in which to perform your contract/release Kegels.

2. Make sure you do not do contract/relax on every exercise, as you will do over 100 Kegels, which is too much for one session! For the other 7 exercises, keep your abdominals contracted at 30% effort and your PFMs relaxed and released.

Overall Considerations for Your Pelvic Pain Pilates Workout

1. Pay attention to your body alignment.

Many exercises require that you keep your back straight and that you sit in good ball posture. Good ball posture is actually the first exercise in the series so you get your body in the right frame of mind before you begin.

2. Pay attention to how you get off the ball.

To get off the ball, roll down until your buttocks are on the floor in order to protect your abdominals. This is especially important if you have diastasis recti of the abdominals. See the next section for information on how to test if you have diastasis recti.

3. Pay attention to your breath.

During the most difficult parts of the exercises, you will be asked to exhale. During the release part of the exercises, you will be asked to inhale.

4. Pay attention to your pelvic floor muscles.

Focus on your PFMs to make sure they are not overly tense and contracted. Whenever possible, incorporate a PFM contraction during exertion and a PFM reverse Kegel release when you return to the start position of the exercise.

5. Start with a warm-up.

Make sure that you begin your workout with a 5 to 10 minute cardio warm-up. You could briskly walk, treadmill, cycle, or any other activity that gets your blood pumping before you begin the routine.

6. Pay attention to your abdomen.

Your abdominals should be moderately engaged throughout the routine. Focus on bringing your belly button to your spine, about 30% of the way. Note that the physio ball exercises work mostly with the transverse abdominal muscles.

Overall Benefits of the Pilates Ball Series

1. Your body will become strong without creating the muscle bulk that lifting traditional weights will do.

2. You will feel more flexible and buoyant, have more energy, and improve joint mobility and range of motion.

3. You will find it easier to remain in a state of good posture.

4. You will have strong abdominals without creating trigger points that are commonly found in females with pelvic pain.

5. You will be better able to discern the overall state of your pelvic floor muscles. The Pilates ball series teaches you how to exercise correctly using both the core muscles and the PFM simultaneously.

Table 5.2: The Herrera Pilates Ball Strengthening Routine for Pelvic Pain™
PDF version of this table available at http://www.RenewPT.com

EXERCISE
1. Seated Ball Posture
2. Seated Ball Marching
3. Arm Circles on Your Back
4. Seated Ball Scapular Squeezes
5. Ball Squats
6. Ball Inner Thigh Squeezes
7. Ball Bridging
8. Alternating Arm and Leg Lifts
9. Ball Plank Side Flutter Kicks
10. Ball Push-Ups

The Herrera Pilates Ball Strengthening Routine for Pelvic Pain™

Seated Ball Posture

WHAT TO DO:

1. Sit tall on the ball with your weight evenly distributed on your sit bones, ears aligned with the shoulders, and abdominal muscles pulled in.

2. Your knees and hips should form a right angle with your feet flat on the floor. It's acceptable for your hips to be slightly higher than your knees, but not the other way around because it will put stress on your lower back and leg muscles.

3. Pull your shoulder blades back towards each other; imagine you are putting your shoulder blades into your back pockets, in and down.

4. Once comfortably in this posture, practice 5 to 10 minutes of diaphragmatic breathing together with reverse Kegels or contract/relax Kegels, depending on where you are in your Kegel program as defined in Chapter 4.

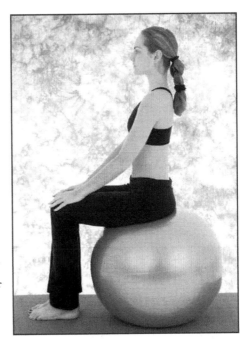

5. This is called "good ball posture" and is the basis of many of the exercises in this series.

WHAT TO WATCH OUT FOR:

1. Incorrect ball size will put increased pressure and strain on muscles. Use Table 5.1 on page 79 to determine which ball is the proper size for your height.

2. Avoid rounding the shoulders or lower back and sticking your chin out, as these will cause pain or strain to your body and could lead to injury.

BENEFITS:

1. Provides good sensory input for the reverse and contract/relax Kegel exercises, as your PFMs are in direct contact with the surface of the ball.

2. Reinforces good sitting posture which will help decrease pain associated with poor sitting and/or slouching at work or home.

Seated Ball Marching

WHAT TO DO:

1. Sit on the center of the ball with good ball posture, with feet hip-width apart and with hands on the ball for added support.

2. Exhale, contract abdominals and PFMs, and then raise the right leg about 2 to 3 inches from the floor. Hold for 2 seconds.

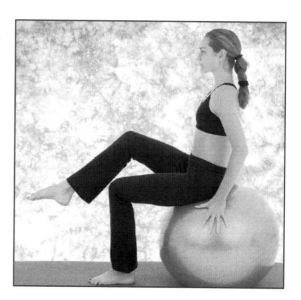

3. Inhale, relax PFMs, and lower the foot. Switch sides, alternating the foot lifts until you have completed 10 repetitions on both sides.

RECOMMENDED STRETCH AFTER THIS EXERCISE:

Ball Warrior Two as detailed in the yoga series in Chapter 6 on page 120.

WHAT TO WATCH OUT FOR:

1. Avoid slouching the lower back and rounding the shoulder blades.

2. Avoid shifting too much weight to the supported foot. Try to keep your weight evenly distributed on your sit bones, hands, and supported foot.

BENEFITS:

1. Strengthens core muscles and leg muscles.

2. Improves balance and posture.

3. Connects you to your PFMs and helps you to contract and relax the pelvic floor muscles.

Arm Circles on Your Back

WHAT TO DO:

1. Sit with good ball posture on the center of the ball.

2. Walk your feet in front of you until your thighs are parallel to the floor and your upper back and head rest comfortably on the ball.

3. Place your arms by the side of your legs, remembering not to collapse into your lower back but keeping the back straight and lifted.

4. Inhale, relax the PFMs, and raise your arms over your head as in the photo.

5. Exhale, contract your PFMs and abdominal muscles, and roll your arms out to the side, finishing with your arms by your legs, creating a circle motion. This is one cycle.

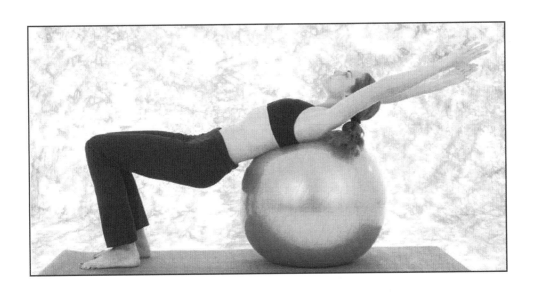

6. Do 10 cycles.

7. When you are finished with this exercise, relax on the floor. Lie down on your back and hug your knees into your chest to release the lower back muscles if they are tight.

RECOMMENDED STRETCH AFTER THIS EXERCISE:

Seated 4 Stretch as detailed in the workplace series in Chapter 7 on page 134. This can be performed on the ball.

WHAT TO WATCH OUT FOR:

1. Avoid slumping in the lower back area. Your lower back should be straight and parallel to your thighs.

2. If your shoulders are too tight to perform the arm circles, skip the circles and extend your arms straight up instead of over your head and then lower them to the side.

3. Keep the shoulder blades pulled together and stabilized on the ball and do not raise them up with the arm circles.

BENEFITS:

1. Strengthens the lower back, gluteal, abdominals, and hamstring muscles.

2. Strengthens the core abdominal muscles and also the arm muscles.

3. Helps improve posture by improving arm range of motion and stretching the chest muscles.

4. Helps to strengthen and relax the pelvic floor muscles.

Seated Ball Scapular Squeezes

WHAT TO DO:

1. Sit with good ball posture with arms reaching forward and palms resting on the front of the thighs.

2. Exhale, contract the abdominals and PFMs, and rotate your palms out. Bring your arms back until your hands are in alignment with the sides of your body.

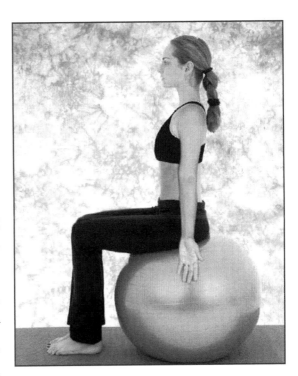

3. Simultaneously bring your shoulder blades towards each other, and imagine them sliding down your back and into your back pockets. Breathe naturally and hold 3 to 5 seconds.

4. Inhale, release the PFM, and rotate your arms and palms back to the start position. Repeat 10 times.

RECOMMENDED STRETCH AFTER THIS EXERCISE:

Seated Side Stretch as detailed in the workplace series in Chapter 7 on page 132.This can also be performed on the physio ball.

WHAT TO WATCH OUT FOR:

1. Avoid slouching the upper and lower back muscles.

2. Do not stick your chin out. Make sure your chin is tucked back at all times.

3. Be sure to keep your chest forward and your shoulder blades back and down.

BENEFITS:

1. Improves posture by strengthening the rhomboideous and lower trap muscles.

2. Encourages PFMs to become toned, strengthened and relaxed.

3. Stretches chest muscles and improves upper body flexibility.

Ball Squats

WHAT TO DO:

1. Place your physio ball against a wall and lean against it with the small of your back touching the ball. Maintain your abdominals slightly engaged with this exercise. Focus on bringing your belly button to your spine, about 30 percent of the effort. Walk your feet forward slightly, allowing your knees to be in a 90-degree angle when you execute the squat.

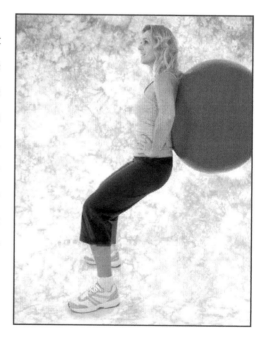

2. Inhale, relax the PFMs, and lower your body until your thighs are parallel to the floor, forming a 90-degree angle. Make sure your knees are on top of your ankles and your back is straight. Hold for 2 to 5 seconds.

3. Exhale, contract your PFMs, and raise yourself to your original position. Repeat 10 times.

RECOMMENDED STRETCH AFTER THIS EXERCISE:

Hamstring on Wall Pose as detailed in the yoga series in Chapter 6 on page 112.

WHAT TO WATCH OUT FOR:

1. Avoid lowering the buttocks lower than the knees, as this will strain your knee ligaments and lower back muscles.

2. Do not let your knees pass your ankles to avoid straining your knees.

3. Watch out for poor breath and PFM coordination.

BENEFITS:

1. Strengthens main muscle groups that become weak in women with pelvic pain, including quadriceps, hamstring, gluteal, inner and outer thigh muscles.

2. Helps maintain correct bio-mechanics because the legs are strong enough to participate in lifting motions.

3. Strengthens and relaxes the PFMs.

Ball Inner Thigh Squeezes

WHAT TO DO:

1. Lie on your left side, with left knee bent and right leg straight up on the ball, as in photo.

2. Exhale, squeeze your abdominals and PFMs, while simultaneously pressing your right leg into the ball for 5 seconds.

3. Inhale, release the downward pressure on the ball from your leg. Then release the PFMs for 5 seconds, and perform a reverse Kegel as outlined in Chapter 4.

4. Repeat 10 times, then switch sides.

RECOMMENDED STRETCH AFTER THIS EXERCISE:

Wall V Stretch as detailed in the yoga series in Chapter 6 on page 111.

WHAT TO WATCH OUT FOR:

1. Be careful to accurately perform the proper contract/relax for your pelvic floor muscles while doing this exercise as you can easily create muscle spasms if the exercise is done incorrectly.

2. Make sure to stretch after this exercise to prevent trigger points in the inner thigh muscles.

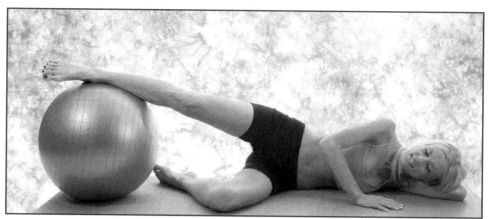

BENEFITS:

1. Tones and strengthens the inner thigh muscles creating balance in the pelvic-hip muscles.

2. Strengthens the PFMs, and can improve leg, foot, ankle and knee alignment for better walking posture.

Ball Bridging

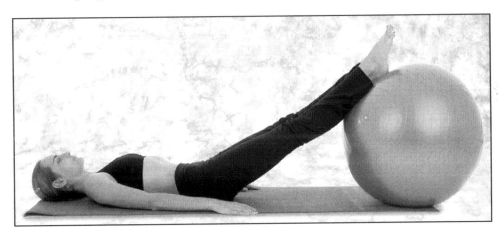

WHAT TO DO:

1. Lie on your back and place your heels on top of the physio ball. Allow your head, shoulders, and arms to relax into the floor.

2. Keeping your legs slightly bent and feet pointing up, exhale and lift your hips up off the floor while simultaneously doing a PFM contraction. Hold this position for 2 to 5 seconds.

3. Inhale and lower your hips slowly while simultaneously performing a reverse Kegel. Hold this position for 5 seconds.

4. Repeat the up and down movement 10 times.

5. If needed, stretch your lower back by gently hugging your knees to your chest.

RECOMMENDED STRETCH AFTER THIS EXERCISE:

Pretzel Pose as detailed in the yoga series in Chapter 6 on page 116.

WHAT TO WATCH OUT FOR:

1. Avoid holding the breath and tensing the shoulders and neck muscles.

2. If you are unable to perform a contract/relax Kegel, focus on the lifting and lowering phase of the bridge.

3. Stop immediately if this exercise produces pain in the lower back or neck muscles.

4. If you experience hamstring soreness, stretch your hamstrings using the Hamstring on Wall Pose found in Chapter 6 on page 112.

BENEFITS:

1. Strengthens core and pelvic floor muscles in addition to the gluteal, hamstrings, and inner thighs.

2. Helps improve lower back spinal alignment.

Alternating Arm and Leg Lifts

WHAT TO DO:

1. Lie on your stomach, facedown on your physio ball, maintaining a good balance between upper and lower body with hands and toes on the floor for added support.

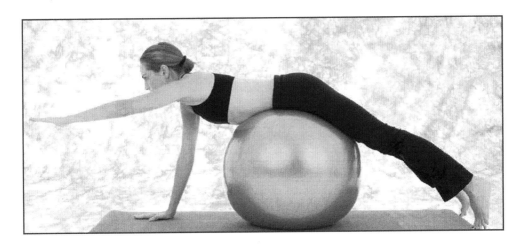

2. Keep hands and feet shoulder-width apart, with your shoulder blades pulled towards each other and your abdominals contracted.

3. Exhale, contract PFMs, and raise your left arm straight out until it is level with your ear.

4. Inhale, relax the PFMs, lower your left arm to the floor, and switch arms. Repeat 10 times on each side.

5. For an additional challenge, raise your right arm and left leg simultaneously. Hold for 2 seconds and then lower both limbs. Repeat with the left arm and right leg.

RECOMMENDED STRETCH AFTER THIS EXERCISE:

Pigeon pose as detailed in the yoga series in Chapter 6 on page 110.

WHAT TO WATCH OUT FOR:

1. The ball will wobble in the beginning as you get used to this exercise. Perform the exercise slowly to help maintain ball stability.

2. Avoid overarching the back and raising the arms and legs too high.

3. Do not raise your hips off the ball as you raise the legs up.

BENEFITS:

1. Strengthens lower back, arms, shoulders, and hip muscles.

2. Improves posture and core strength.

3. Improves PFM strength, relaxation, and coordination.

Ball Plank Side Flutter Kicks

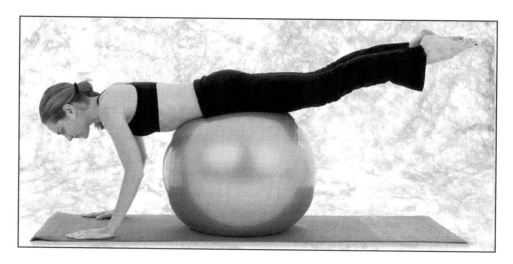

WHAT TO DO:

1. Lie on your stomach, facedown on your physio ball with palms resting on the floor.

2. Walk your hands and body forward until the ball is at your upper thighs. Make sure to keep your hands a little wider than shoulder-width apart and your feet together.

3. Exhale, contract the PFMs and abdominals, and bring your legs out to the side a little wider than hip-width apart for 3 to 5 seconds. Be careful not to hyper-extend or round your back.

4. Inhale, release the PFMs, and bring your legs back to starting position. Relax for 3 to 5 seconds, then repeat 10 times.

5. For an extra challenge, add a Dyna-Band around your ankles to make the outward movement of your legs more difficult. A Dyna-Band is an elastic band with different color-coded resistance. Start with the easiest resistance and progress as tolerated.

RECOMMENDED STRETCH AFTER THIS EXERCISE:

Knee Down Twist pose as detailed in the yoga series in Chapter 6 on page 108.

WHAT TO WATCH OUT FOR:

1. Avoid hyper-extending your elbows, which will put strain and stress on the ligaments.

2. Keep your neck in alignment with the rest of your spine and avoid sticking your jaw out.

3. Avoid sagging in the lower back which could potentially hurt your spine.

4. Be careful of wrist and hand pain.

BENEFITS:

1. Strengthens the outer thighs, gluteal muscles, arms and shoulders.

2. Improves core and PFM strength, relaxation and coordination.

Ball Push-Ups

WHAT TO DO:

1. Lie on your stomach, facedown on your physio ball with palms resting on the floor.

2. Walk your hands and body forward until the ball is at your shins, as in the photo below. Make sure to keep your feet together and your hands a little wider than shoulder-width apart. To make it a bit easier, only walk your body forward to your upper thighs.

3. Inhale, relax the PFMs, bend your arms and lower your body until your elbows are aligned with your shoulders, making a right angle.

4. Exhale, contract the PFMs and abdominals, and straighten out the arms and elbows without hyper-extending the elbows. Repeat 10 times.

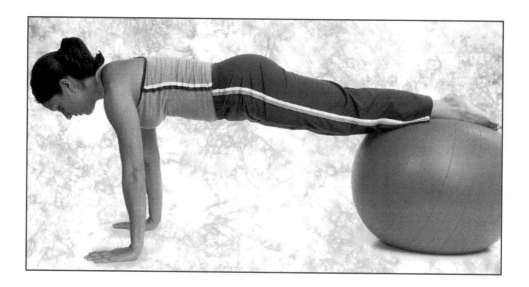

RECOMMENDED STRETCH AFTER THIS EXERCISE:

Seated Chest Opener as detailed in the workplace series in Chapter 7 on page 139. This can be performed on the physio ball.

WHAT TO WATCH OUT FOR:

1. If it is too difficult to lower your body all the way, do baby push-ups by not lowering the body too much.

2. Avoid hyper-extending your elbows, which will put strain and stress on the ligaments.

3. Keep your neck in alignment with the rest of your spine and avoid sticking your jaw out.

4. Avoid sagging in the lower back which could potentially hurt your spine.

5. Be careful of wrist and hand pain. Keep your body weight evenly distributed among all 5 fingers and imagine that you are pushing the floor away from you as you raise your body up.

BENEFITS:

1. Strengthens the chest and increases the endurance of the shoulders and arm muscles.

2. Improves core and PFM strength.

Now that you have become familiar with the key aspects of the strengthening series, let's take a look at the yoga series in the next chapter, which is the perfect complement to your conditioning program.

Chapter Six

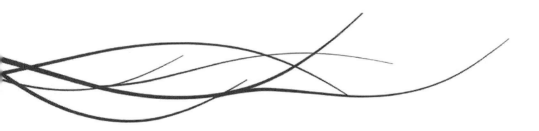

*"You may encounter many defeats, but you must not be defeated.
In fact, it may be necessary to encounter the defeats,
so you can know who you are, what you can rise from,
and how you can still come out of it."*
— Maya Angelou

Chapter 6

THE HERRERA YOGA SERIES FOR PELVIC PAIN™

The essential stretches highlighted in this chapter help stretch the outer pelvic hip muscles, the lower back, the gluteal muscles and abdominal muscles, all of which are intimately connected with your PFMs. By stretching these adjacent, outer pelvic and hip muscles, you are indirectly releasing tension in the PFMs. The poses in this yoga series were chosen because I found that when these were incorporated into their treatment programs, my patients felt less overall pain and the yoga series helped control the intensity of their flare-ups. My patients tell me that when they have painful flare-ups, this yoga series is a lifesaver. Many of my patients have also told me that the stretching helped to release the tension and tightness they feel in their pelvic, lower back and hip muscles.

The series also indirectly helps you feel more relaxed and calm. Many patients also report that after consistently performing the yoga series they are able to insert their dilators more easily and perform their intravaginal stretching, trigger point and myofascial releases with less difficulty and with less pain. Do not worry if you have not done yoga before. The series can be performed by most women even if stretching is entirely new. Remember to be content to "be" just where you are that day, not allowing yourself to get discouraged if you discover an extremely difficult and painful stretch.

When my patients perform the stretching poses highlighted in this chapter while hooked up to computerized biofeedback sensors, their pelvic floor muscle resting baseline outputs are reduced. The resting baseline seen with biofeedback represents the activity in the pelvic floor muscles at rest. At rest, the baseline should appear flat, smooth and should register under two microvolts. But in women with sexual and pelvic pain, resting biofeedback levels are often erratic and tremendously higher than two microvolts. I frequently use biofeedback as a tool to treat sexual pain and pelvic pain because it allows my patients to visualize muscles that are difficult to see, allowing them to tune in to these areas.

The exercises in this chapter are yoga-based. I recommend that they be performed in sequential order; these poses were written in this order so that you can flow into and out of the poses with ease. However, once you have mastered the series, you can perform just the poses that give you the most pain relief. Think of it as your own vaginal pelvic yoga class.

While performing the exercises, always stay in tune with your pelvic floor muscles. Ask yourself, "Do my pelvic floor muscles feel uptight or relaxed and loose?" With all the stretches, you should keep your focus on maintaining relaxed and released PFMs. Many of the stretches in this chapter are intense and may cause you pain while you are performing them. Try to perform the stretches only to the point where you feel a mild stretch. Stretching too vigorously can lead to an increase in muscle soreness and can increase the tension in the pelvic floor muscles, resulting in heightened pelvic pain. Keep your mind focused on the stretches and do not let your mind wander to what you have to do today at work or what chores you need to do. It is important to stay connected with all the sensations you are feeling and especially important to avoid holding your breath. Holding your breath, also called valsalva, will strain and excessively stress your pelvic floor muscles.

Let this stretching series become an integral part of your transformational body work, and you will feel better both physically and mentally afterwards.

The Herrera Yoga Series Program Guidelines

1. All stretches should be held for 10 to 60 seconds depending on your tolerance and pain.

2. The basic yoga core series should be done in its entirety as you become accustomed to the moves. As you get more used to the series, you can choose parts that are more effective for your particular needs and customize your program.

3. For better results and for pain reduction it is best to perform the yoga series up to three times per week (e.g., Monday, Wednesday, and Friday).

4. While performing the series, practice Tension Release Breathing or TRB. To understand TRB in your mind's eye, send your in-breath or inhalation to the part of your muscles where you feel the most tension or pain. Imagine that you are collecting the tension in your muscles with your in-breath. With your out-breath, exhale all the tension out of the muscles. You will learn to relax and ease the tension in your muscles much easier by performing the stretches with proper breathing techniques. I find that the patients who use this type of breathing with their stretching are able to control their pain better, especially during muscle flare-ups.

5. Make the length of your inhalation breath equal to the length of your exhalation. For instance breathe in for a count of 4 and exhale for a count of 4.

6. Try to release your PFM while you inhale. This may seem counterintuitive at first, but by doing this you will actually be working with the natural rhythm of the organs when breathing. Upon inhalation, the diaphragm drops down naturally, so try to let the PFM release as well. My patients typically have some difficulty mastering this release technique, so don't worry if this happens to you. The important thing is to focus on the PFM. If you can get a release with the exhale only at first, this is fine as well.

7. Never go beyond the stretching limit of your muscles. You should feel a mild stretch while in the poses. Stretching too deeply can lead to muscle strain, micro-tears, muscle pulls, and joint problems. All stretches are static and require that you hold them at the end position without moving. Never bounce in the stretch as you could pull or strain a muscle. This is called ballistic stretching, and it is not recommended for women suffering from pelvic pain.

8. Always get out of your stretches mindfully and slowly.

9. Start with the complete core series at first to help you gain confidence. You can then customize your poses to enhance your healing. If there are muscles that feel tighter and more tense, focus your energy on stretches that target that particular muscle.

10. For women who are inflexible or who have never stretched on a regular basis, I recommend that you hold the poses for less time until you build up your momentum.

11. The key is to pay attention to your body and observe the sensations created in your body during your yoga practice. Stay in the moment with all stretching exercises.

12. The last 4 poses of the yoga series require a a physio ball. See Chapter 5, page 79 for details on how to purchase a physio ball for your body type.

Table 6.1: The Herrera Yoga Series for Pelvic Pain™ Pose Flow Chart
PDF version of this table available at http://www.Renew-PT.com

NAME OF POSE OR STRETCH
1. Corpse Pose (start)
2. Goddess Pose
3. Knee Down Twist
4. Pigeon
5. Wall V Stretch
6. Hamstring on Wall Pose
7. Mermaid Stretch
8. Ankle to Knee
9. Pretzel Pose
10. Z Stretch
11. Ball Wheel
12. Warrior Two on Ball
13. Ball Child's Pose
14. Prayer Squat
15. Corpse Pose (end)

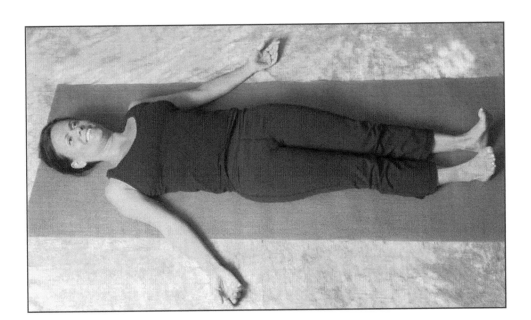

Corpse Pose

WHAT TO DO:

1. Lie on your back with your legs straight and arms relaxed out to the side, palms facing up. Feel your belly rise gently when you inhale and feel your belly lower when you exhale.

2. Now bring your awareness to your PFMs and direct your inhalation into this area. With your mind's eye, see and feel your PFMs let go and release as you breathe in. When you exhale, release the stress, tension and pain held in the body.

3. If your mind wanders, say the word *release* and bring your awareness back to your breathing.

4. Practice your reverse Kegels in this pose as outlined in Chapter 4, page 61.

WHAT TO WATCH OUT FOR:

1. Be careful not to hold your breath and do not push the muscles out.

2. If you cannot release the PFMs when you inhale, do not worry. You can also focus on PFM release on the exhale until you have learned to release them on the inhale. Remember, your diaphragm goes down on the in-breath, so focus on dropping the PFMs in conjunction with your diaphragm.

BENEFITS:

1. Reduces pelvic/vaginal muscle tension.

2. Relieves pelvic pain.

3. Reduces stress.

4. Quiets the mind.

5. Stretches inner thigh/groin muscles which are intimately connected to the PFM.

Goddess Pose

WHAT TO DO:

1. Lie on your back and place the soles of your feet together. Allow the weight of your legs to pull your knees toward the floor.

2. You will feel a gentle stretch and release on your inner thigh muscles.

3. Breathe diaphragmatically as you feel your inner thigh muscles release. This is also a great pose in which to practice your daily meditation and reverse Kegels.

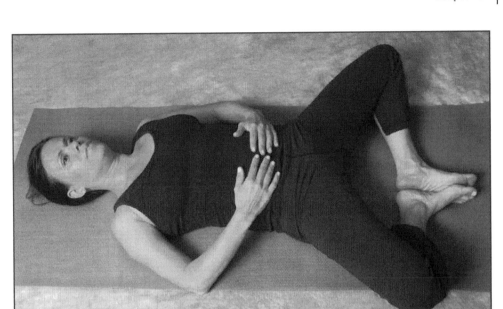

WHAT TO WATCH OUT FOR:

1. Strain on the inner thighs will be felt by women with tight muscles in this area. To make this exercise more comfortable, if you are feeling excessive strain or pain, place one to two pillows under each knee for added support.

2. If you experience discomfort in the sacroiliac joint or lower back area, place one to two pillows under your knees for added support and to reduce stress in the lower back.

BENEFITS:

1. Inner thigh muscles are frequently tight in women with pelvic pain and are often filled with trigger points that can refer pain to the pelvic floor and even elicit symptoms of urinary urgency. This intimate relationship is sometimes overlooked but these important muscles can actually contribute to overall pelvic misalignment.

2. The Goddess Pose is a great stress-releasing position to do your trigger

point releases and to massage the groin, inner thigh, and labias. This pose is also good for external PFM stretching, as highlighted in Part III of this book.

Knee Down Twist

WHAT TO DO:

1. Lie on your back and grab your right knee with your left hand, keeping your right hand extended out to the side as in the photo. Gently bring your right knee across your body until the right knee makes contact with the floor, if possible.

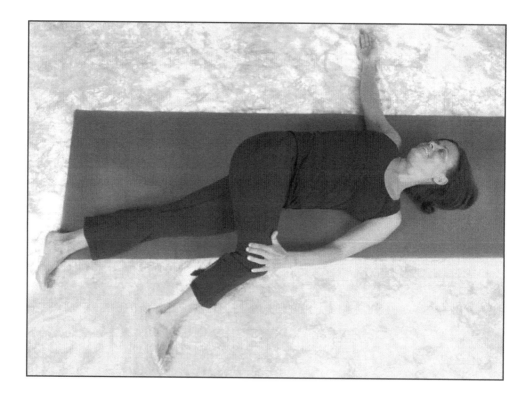

2. Your lower back will come off the floor, creating a spinal twisting motion. Focus your gaze on your outstretched right hand.

3. You may hear or feel a spinal release, as this pose can elicit a gentle spinal adjustment.

4. Repeat on the other side.

WHAT TO WATCH OUT FOR:

1. Avoid pulling the leg across the body too vigorously and creating nerve pain and or lower back pain.

2. Do not hold your breath as this is an intense stretch.

3. If you experience excessive pain in your lower back muscles or tailbone, you might be forcing the knee down to the floor too hard. Your lumbar spine may also have restrictions and you may find that this stretch is not appropriate for you in the beginning.

4. If you feel pain traveling down the leg, stop immediately.

BENEFITS:

1. Enhances proper nerve function and blood supply for a healthier vagina, rectum, and pelvic muscles.

2. The twisting motion compresses your organs, so when you release the pose, fresh blood and energy flows into your organs.

3. Helps decrease pelvic congestion.

Pigeon

WHAT TO DO:

1. Get on all fours with your knees below your hips and your hands underneath your shoulders.

2. Bring the left knee forward until it touches the right wrist; keep the left leg straight back behind you.

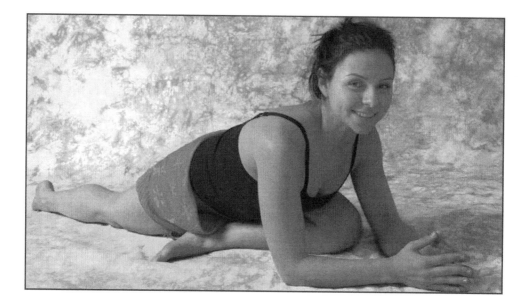

3. Try to move your right foot until it is directly below your left hip. If this is not possible, keep the foot back.

4. Keep your hips squared and level.

5. With your arms straight, support your torso. If you are very flexible, support your torso while resting on your elbows.

6. Keep your gaze straight ahead. If you are resting on your elbows, you can drop the head down.

7. Use a folded blanket or pillow under your right buttock if you have trouble lowering the hips evenly.

8. Switch sides and repeat.

WHAT TO WATCH OUT FOR:

1. Do not force yourself into this pose as it will strain your knees and hips.

2. Avoid tensing the pelvic floor muscles while in this pose.

BENEFITS:

1. Opens up the hip flexors and hip rotators which are commonly tight in women with pelvic pain.

2. Promotes hip and lower back flexibility.

Wall V Stretch

WHAT TO DO:

1. Lie face up near a wall with your buttocks as close to the wall as possible, and your legs up the wall.

2. Keep your hips and lower back flat on the floor.

3. Keep your body relaxed while you move both feet apart from each other.

4. Only open your legs until you feel a mild to medium stretch in your inner thigh muscles.

WHAT TO WATCH OUT FOR:

1. Avoid pulling the legs apart with too much force as this could lead to an inner-groin or leg muscle pull or strain. Keep this stretch gentle and avoid

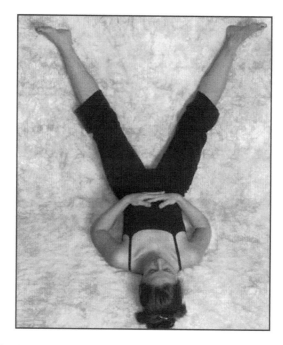

pulling the thighs out too vigorously which can create pain with the stretch.

2. Many times pain during this stretch can translate to more tension in the pelvic floor muscles. It is extremely important to be aware of any increased tension in the PFMs and to release it while performing this stretch.

BENEFITS:

1. Increases flexibility in the inner thigh muscles and creates an overflow releasing effect to the pelvic floor muscles.

2. Indirectly helps to stretch out the skin and any scar present in the perineum, enhancing scar mobility.

Hamstring on Wall Pose
WHAT TO DO:

1. Lie face up near a wall with your buttocks facing the wall.

2. Place your hands under your knees and bring your knees to your chest. Pause here if needed for a nice lower back stretch.

3. Scoot your buttocks as close to the wall as possible.

4. Straighten out your left leg against the wall while maintaining the right leg bent against your chest.

5. Straigthen the right knee until a stretch is felt in the hamstring muscle.

6. Hold and then repeat on the other side.

WHAT TO WATCH OUT FOR:

1. Avoid straightening the knee with too much vigor and force as this can result in lower back pain or a micro-tear of the hamstring muscle.

2. Prevent your lower back from overarching. Keep your lumbar spine flat against the floor.

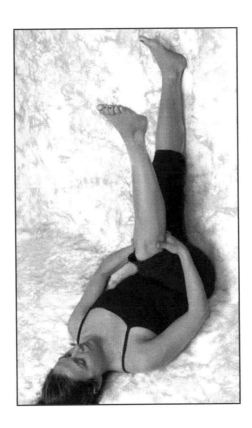

BENEFITS:

1. Stretching the hamstring muscle helps keep the pelvis in good alignment and improve posture.

2. Helps prevent lower back pain and excessive tension in the hips, pelvis and PFM.

3. Helps stretch out the area through which the pudendal, sciatic, and obturator nerve travel. These nerves are important for PFM health, pelvic sensation, and pelvic motion.

Mermaid Stretch

WHAT TO DO:

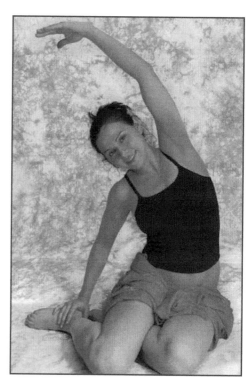

1. Sit with both legs bent to the right side and hold on to the top leg, as in the photo.

2. Lift the left arm upwards and gently bend to the right side until a stretch is felt in the left side muscles.

3. Hold and then repeat on the other side.

WHAT TO WATCH OUT FOR:

1. Imagine your outstretched arm touching the ceiling before you reach over.

2. Avoid compressing into the sides as this can cause pain in the lower back and side muscles.

BENEFITS:

1. Stretches the side muscles, including the quadratus lumborum or QL, latissimus dorsi, and intercostal muscles, while simultaneously improving spinal movement.

2. Improves nerve function and creates better rib mobility, enhancing diaphragmatic breathing.

Ankle to Knee

WHAT TO DO:

1. Sit tall on your sit bones and place your right ankle slightly off your left knee and place your left ankle under your right knee as in photo.

2. If you cannot get your legs to create two right angles, don't worry; slide your lower leg towards your buttocks.

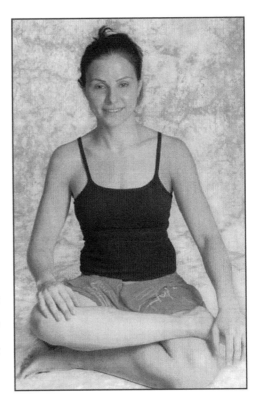

3. Keeping your back straight, try to walk your fingertips forward.

4. To advance the pose, reach up and over with your right hand.

5. Repeat, crossing your legs the other way.

6. You may feel an intense stretch in the gluteal muscles of your top leg. Listen to your body, modify first and then consider getting out of the pose if the pain is too much.

7. To take it a step further, send your in-breath to the place in your hips that you feel the most tension and with your out-breath release the tension out of the hips.

8. For fantastic pain relief, massage the gluteal muscles of your top leg with your hands while in this pose.

WHAT TO WATCH OUT FOR:

1. Stay in a pain-free range as this is a difficult stretch that can cause some stretching pain. Staying within a pain-free range will avoid overflowing the tension to your hips.

2. Avoid holding your breath.

3. Put a small folded towel under your lower ankle if there is pain.

4. Make sure to keep both sit bones on the floor and equally distribute your weight on them.

BENEFITS:

This stretch completely opens up the hips and gluteal muscles. By increasing the flexibility of your hips, you get better blood flow to the pelvic organs and you will also enhance nerve function.

Pretzel Pose

WHAT TO DO:

1. Sit tall on your sit bones with your back straight.

2. Place the right knee over the left knee as in photo.

3. Keeping your back straight, try to walk your fingertips forward.

4. To advance the pose, reach up and over with your right hand.

5. Repeat, crossing your legs the other way.

WHAT TO WATCH OUT FOR:

1. Keep your back straight.

2. Sit high on your sit bones and keep your weight evenly distributed on both buttock cheeks.

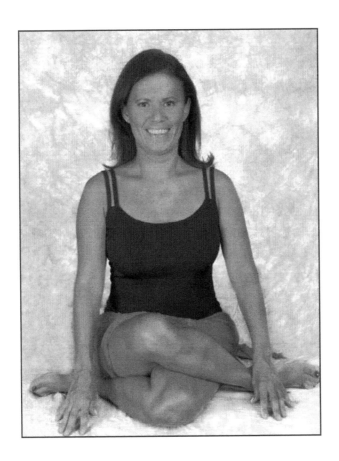

3. Don't hold your breath.

BENEFITS:

1. Helps eliminate spasms and trigger points in the hip muscles.

2. Increases hip flexibility.

Z Stretch

WHAT TO DO:

1. Sit with the soles of your feet together, and then bring the right leg behind you, keeping your left leg in the same position. Your legs will create a "Z" shape.

2. Place your palms gently on your knees, focusing on keeping your back straight.

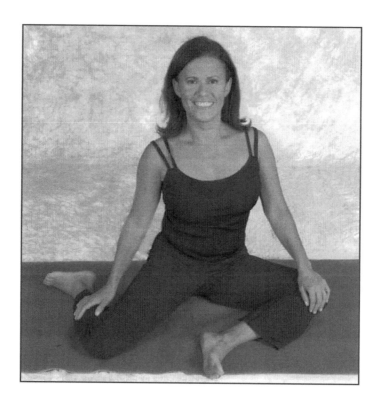

3. Switch sides and repeat.

WHAT TO WATCH OUT FOR:

If you experience knee or hip pain, bring the back leg forward.

BENEFITS:

1. Stretches hips, groin, and inner thigh muscles.

2. Improves postural alignment, helping your body maintain erect posture.

Ball Wheel

WHAT TO DO:

1. Lie with your back flat on the ball and walk your body back until the palms of your hands are directly behind you on the floor, as in the photo.

2. If this position is too intense, modify it so that you do not put your palms on the floor. Just roll back until you stretch in your abdominals, chest, and

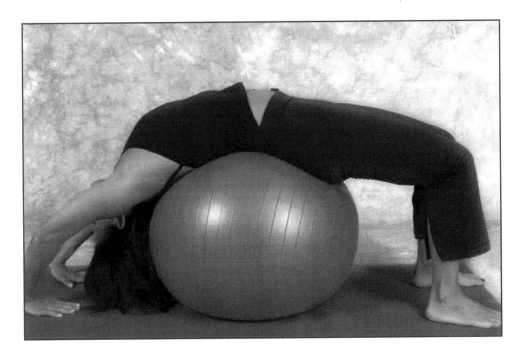

throughout the front of your body.

WHAT TO WATCH OUT FOR:

This is a very intense position. If your back does not have the flexibility to get into this pose, be gentle with yourself. Over time this pose will help relieve your stress and calm your mind in addition to being a great stretch

BENEFITS:

1. Serves as a great stress reliever.

2. Opens up muscles which become tight due to chronic poor posture and slouching.

Warrior Two on Ball

WHAT TO DO:

1. Place physio ball under your buttocks for support.

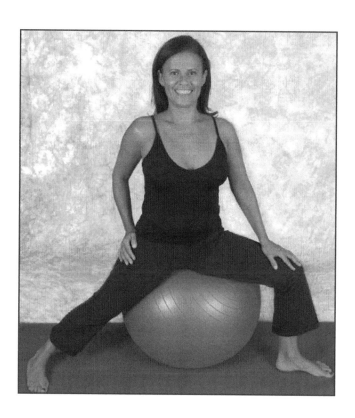

2. Bring your feet about 3 to 4 feet apart.

3. Turn your left foot out to open up the left leg, so that the left knee is over the ankle.

4. Rotate your right foot in slightly to create a 45-degree angle between your left and right foot. These angles can vary depending on the flexibility of your hips.

5. Inhale, raise your arms out to the side and look over your left shoulder. Keeping your shoulders and hips facing forward, externally rotate your hips open until you feel a stretch in your hips, inner thighs, and groin. Hold, breathe several cycles and then switch sides.

WHAT TO WATCH OUT FOR:

1. Avoid allowing your bent knee to go past 90 degrees, which would allow your knees to go past your toes as this can create knee pain and strain the knee ligaments.

2. Avoid leaning backwards and putting stress on the lower back muscles.

BENEFITS:

1. Opens up the anterior hip, through which pelvic blood supply and nerves travel, increasing blood flow and improving nerve function.

2. Increases the flexibility of the groin, hips, and inner thigh muscles.

3. Helps relieve back pain, improves balance and strengthens the legs.

Ball Child's Pose

WHAT TO DO:

1. Get onto your hands and knees with pointed toes. Bring your buttocks towards your heels, lowering your chest towards the floor.

2. Place your hands outstretched on the ball as in the photo.

3. If this stretch is too intense, place your hands next to your body with palms up.

4. For a deeper stretch, gently roll your outstretched arms and trunk to the right, then to the left, then to neutral, using the ball to guide your motion. This is called the Angled Child's Pose.

WHAT TO WATCH OUT FOR:

1. If you feel pain in the ankles, use a pillow under your feet.

2. If your chest cannot reach the floor or you have pain or discomfort, fold a blanket or towel and place this between your buttocks and legs to give yourself additional support.

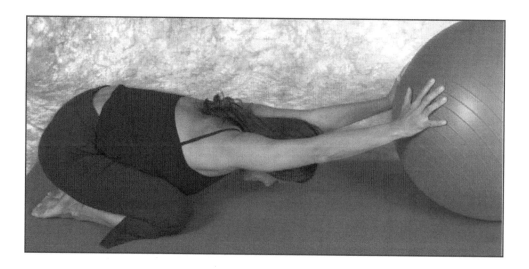

3. If you have preexisting knee conditions and experience pain in the knees with this pose, try the blanket and towel. If the pain persists, this pose might not be appropriate for you.

BENEFITS:

1. Stretches hips, ankles, and thighs.

2. Relieves neck and lower back pain.

3. Relieves stress by calming down the brain.

Prayer Squat

WHAT TO DO:

1. Adopt a squatting position as in the photo.

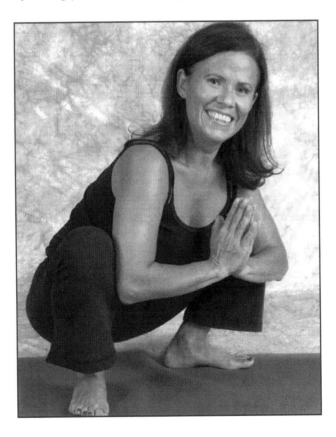

2. Place your arm across your chest in prayer position.

3. Breathe diaphragmatically and hold the prayer position for 10 to 60 seconds.

4. As tolerated, use your arms to press your legs apart

5. Focus on releasing your pelvic floor muscles.

WHAT TO WATCH OUT FOR:

1. This can be a very stressful position for women who lack flexibility in the hips and calves.

2. To make the Prayer Pose easier, put some pillows under your feet. You can also do the Prayer Pose against the wall for back support. It might also be helpful to place a pillow underneath the buttocks to take pressure off the body and to make the Prayer Pose easier to handle.

BENEFITS:

1. Opens up the hips, leg and calf muscles.

2 Stretches the calf, back and hip muscles. Because the PFMs are naturally relaxed in this position, it is a great position to use during painful flare-ups.

3. Relieves back pain and hip pain.

You have now been introduced to two of the pillars of your program's foundation, the strengthening and stretching series. Now let's be sure to cover our bases while at the workplace, where we will spend about 40 percent of our time during the weekdays.

Chapter Seven

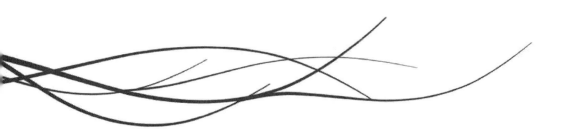

"You must find the place inside yourself where
nothing is impossible."
— Deepak Chopra

Chapter 7

STRETCHING AT THE WORKPLACE

I always remember as a child being told that sitting up straight was something very important for me to do. My second-grade teacher would give gold stars to the children who sat upright and tall in their chairs and even a small gift to the child who collected the most stars. This positive reinforcement has remained instilled in me to this day and is a concept that has absolute relevance for my current line of work in treating pelvic pain. Most women with pelvic pain have postural issues as a contributing factor because certain muscles have become inflexible and weak, leading to poor sitting, standing, and walking posture. Sometimes poor posture comes about as a protective mechanism, as women draw inward into their bodies in response to pain and feelings of hopelessness. Women who tell me they want to shut off from the world because their pain has overtaken their lives often assume postures that are hunched over or slouched. Good posture is one of the keys to starting on the road of taking control over your pain. The mind will begin to follow the body if you correct the way you carry yourself. With correct posture you will feel better, think better, and become more confident and reassured about yourself.

The women I treat often sit with poor posture between 6 to 10 hours a day while on the job. By the end of their workday, they complain about various pains and discomforts in the vulva, rectal area, hips, and low back. They find that sitting for any period of time is unbearable, and many grow to dread their jobs for this reason. They report feeling a deep burning sensation from constant pressure on the perineum, a deep ache in their vaginas, or general pain and aches in the hips. They say getting through their workday is sometimes impossible, and many call in sick during their flare-ups, missing workdays and even missing pay.

In these cases, I try to build up their sitting tolerance and give them stretches and pain-relieving strategies they can do at their job. Since bad workplace posture is so prevalent amongst my patients, I have included discreet pain relieving and stress-reducing techniques in *Ending Female Pain*. The stretches can be performed throughout the day. The longer your workday is, the more frequently you should do them. For a typical 8-hour day you should perform the stretches at least 1 to 3 times. Of course if you do these stretches constantly throughout your workday you will achieve greater flexibility, less muscular tension and less sitting pain. Being mindful of your posture can also subliminally contribute to giving you a positive attitude, as you hold your body strong and let your mind know you are not giving up.

Besides the stretches highlighted in this chapter it is extremely important to have your computer workstation set up properly following ergonomic principles. When a patient comes to see me I always ask one critical thing, "What type of job do you do?" This question is key because a poor work environment can be a contributing factor or even a root cause of pain. I also ask, "Has your station been evaluated for proper ergonomics?" The answer from most patients is no. Day after day of bad posture at work contributes to excess strain and stress on the lower back, the pelvic floor muscles, hip muscles, and gluteal muscles.

Many corporate environments have a specialist on staff that will evaluate and correct your workstation environment. If you have a resource like this at your job, use it. Otherwise follow the basic guidelines recommended in this book to check your own work area. There are four areas of focus for a proper set-up: the monitor, the chair, the mouse and the lighting. To set up your computer station correctly and to maintain a healthier work environment make sure your work area adheres to the recommendations listed in Table 7.1. From my personal experience, making the smallest adjustment to your desk environment can make a huge difference to your posture and improve your level of comfort while sitting.

Table: 7.1: Suggestions for a Healthier Work Environment and Proper Computer Ergonomics

WORK CONSIDERATIONS TO REDUCE PELVIC PAIN
1. Position your monitor directly in front of you. You should be able to comfortably view the screen without having to tilt your neck backwards or forwards. A good rule of thumb is that the top of your monitor should be aligned with your forehead and your eyes level to the screen.
2. Your back should be completely supported and straight. Avoid slumping and slouching to prevent straining the lower back and hip muscles. It is essential that you purchase a lumbar roll if your chair does not provide lumbar support. A lumbar roll will help maintain a neutral spine.
3. Make sure to keep your feet flat on the floor. Use a foot stool if necessary. Your upper thighs should be parallel to the floor. Avoid crossing your legs under the chair.
4. Keep elbows at right angles with forearms parallel to the floor. Also keep wrist in a neutral, or flat and straight position.
5. Never hold the phone between your head and shoulder. Use head phones to avoid putting excessive stress on the neck and upper back muscles.
6. Avoid overreaching for the mouse. Your mouse should be near your keyboard.
7. Purchase a good chair. The proper chair has a backrest that can be adjusted. It's best to have the back of the chair incline slightly backwards. This has the effect of relaxing the spinal musculature and decreasing spinal pressure. You can also choose to have the back rest directly upright.
8. Avoid having the monitor too close to your eyes. Recommended distance is from 20 to 25 inches.
9. Avoid storing work-related materials and files below your desk and workstation which can lead to excessive bending, putting unnecessary stress on the back and hip muscles.
10. Take frequent breaks, at least 5 to 10 minutes every hour. While on your breaks do your stretches and releasing exercises.

Now that your computer and work area are optimally aligned and safe for good posture, you need to pay attention to your sitting posture while at your workstation. Correct sitting posture is easy. What's hard for most individuals is to stay within that posture throughout their workday. It is easy to sit in a slumped, forward-head position, but this only contributes to more muscular weakness and pain. For optimal sitting posture follow the recommendations listed in Table 7.2.

Table 7.2: Optimal Sitting Posture for Work and for Exercising on the Job

SPECIAL POSTURE CONSIDERATIONS AT THE WORKPLACE
1. When sitting, maintain a neutral spine at all times. Keep your back straight, knees bent, and head centered over your shoulders. Avoid slouching even though it may feel good at the time. Slouching eventually overstretches spinal ligaments and muscles, creating a vicious cycle oftentimes causing pain.
2. Avoid hiking up or rounding your shoulders while sitting. Shoulders should be relaxed and should drape flat over your ribs.
3. Sit back into the chair so your back is totally supported. Avoid sitting at the front of your chair where you may end up slouching.
4. Your pelvis should be neutral. Avoid rounding the lower back while you are sitting, which adversely affects the nerves that innervate the pelvic muscles and creates excessive stress on your hips and PFM.
5. Don't let your jaw stick out. Align your head with your shoulders and pelvis, and tuck in your chin.
6. Take frequent breaks and avoid sitting for longer than 45 minutes at a time.
7. Keep your feet flat on the floor. Get a stool if needed.

My patients tell me they love their work stretches. They say that their pain is much less at the end of the day; they function better and are able to control pain levels while at work more easily. The following work stretches should be performed at least 1 to 3 times daily or if needed. All stretches are to be performed in a pain-free range and don y until you feel a gentle stretch in the muscles. Make sure to read the gene idelines found in Table 7.3 and to apply them to all of the stretches in the

Table 7.3: Seated Stretch General Guidelines

SPECIAL POSTURE CONSIDERATIONS AT THE WORKPLACE
1. Always use Tension Releasing Breathing, or TRB, while holding stretches. Never hold your breath.
2. Never bounce while holding a stretch.
3. Hold the stretch for as long as tolerated, usually anywhere from 10 seconds to 1 minute.
4. Many of the stretches require that you sit at the front edge of the chair. Always use correct seated posture as described above when not doing the stretch.
5. Always pay attention to your pelvic floor muscles and avoid holding tension in them as you stretch.

Herrera Workplace Stretching Series for Pelvic Pain

Table 7.4: Workplace Stretching Series for Pelvic Pain

Frequency –Monday to Friday

NAME OF STRETCH
1. Seated Half-Wind
2. Seated Side Stretch
3. Seated 4 Stretch
4. Seated Spinal Twist
5. Seated Thigh Release
6. Seated Chest Opener
7. Seated Reverse Kegels
8. Seated Diaphragmatic Breathing

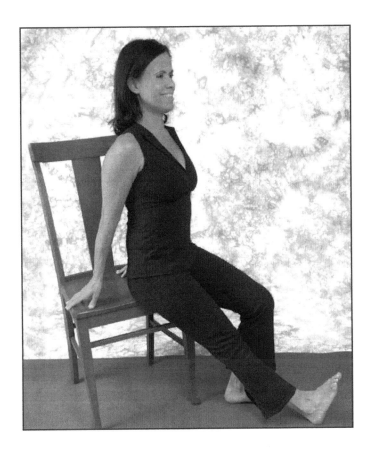

Seated Half-Wind

WHAT TO DO:

1. Adopt a good seated posture at the edge of your seat.

2. Straighten out your right leg and point your toes towards your head until you feel a stretch behind the back of your leg and calf.

3. For deeper stretching, bend forward from the hips while keeping your back straight and shoulders square.

4. Switch legs and repeat.

WHAT TO WATCH OUT FOR:

1. Watch out for pain radiating into the toes. If this occurs, stretch less aggressively, keeping the foot in a more neutral position instead of pointing it up. Stop immediately if pain persists despite modification.

2. If you experience pain or discomfort in the lower back, make sure you remain upright instead of leaning forward. If pain continues in the lower back muscles, stop.

3. Poor postural alignment while doing this stretch can put excessive strain on your upper and lower back muscles. Make sure you don't overarch your back as well.

BENEFITS:

1. This stretch improves hamstring and calf flexibility.

2. Relieves tension in pelvic floor muscles via fascial connections throughout the hamstrings.

3. Helps to decrease lower back pain encouraging good posture and pelvic/ hip alignment.

Seated Side Stretch

WHAT TO DO:

1. Start in a seated position at the front of your chair, using good posture as outlined earlier in the chapter.

2. Raise your right arm up towards ceiling and place your left arm at your hips.

3. Bend your upper body to the left while reaching up and over with your right arm.

4. Bring your body back to the center and repeat the pose on the other side.

WHAT TO WATCH OUT FOR:

1. Avoid compressing into the left side. Think tall as you bend sideways.

2. Avoid overstretching and forcing the side-bend as this can cause pain to the intercostals or side muscles.

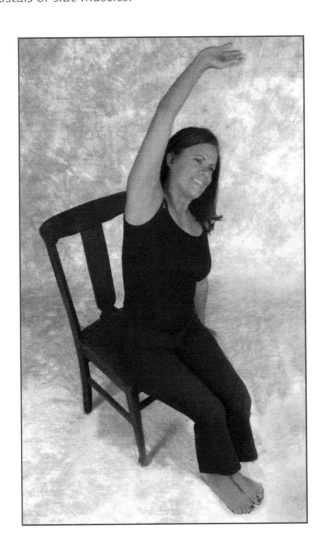

BENEFITS:

1. Helps increase the flexibility of your spine, arms, and rib cage.

2. Helps to realign pelvic bones and maintain lumbar spine and sacral alignment.

3. Enhances nerve function.

4. Facilitates rib expansion which will help get more oxygen into your lungs and promote better breathing.

Seated 4 Stretch

WHAT TO DO:

1. While seated in good posture at the edge of your seat, place the left ankle lightly on the thigh of the right leg making a figure 4. Keep your hips square, your shoulders down and back as you sit straight.

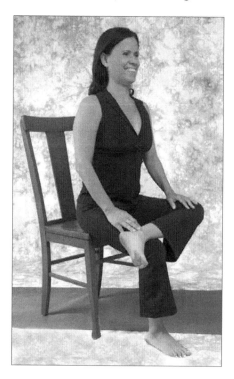

2. If you are able, gently press your crossed leg down but not lower than your thigh.

3. For a deeper stretch, lean forward from the hips with a straight back. For an even deeper stretch rotate your upper body slightly towards your feet.

4. Bring your body back to center and repeat the pose on the other side.

WHAT TO WATCH OUT FOR:

1. Don't torque the ankle bone. Remember to keep the ankle bone slightly off the resting thigh to avoid stressing it.

2. Avoid slouching in this posture to prevent stress on the lumbar spinal nerves and to make this stretch more effective.

3. If your pain increases and/or radiates into your thigh or lower leg/foot, or persists for 30 minutes or longer, discontinue this stretch and consult your healthcare professional.

BENEFITS:

1. Helps prevent sciatica.

2. Helps to stretch the piriformis muscle and maintain pelvic alignment.

3. Helps increase the mobility and function of the major nerve roots of the lumbar and sacral spine which innervate the pelvic floor muscles and internal pelvic organs.

4. Improves blood flow to the hip and pelvic muscles.

Seated Spinal Twist

WHAT TO DO:

1. Sit at the edge of your seat and cross your right thigh over your left thigh. Place your left hand on your right knee and gently pull the knee across the body.

2. Place your right hand behind you, open up the chest and lengthen your spine upward, bringing your gaze over your right shoulder while simultaneously twisting.

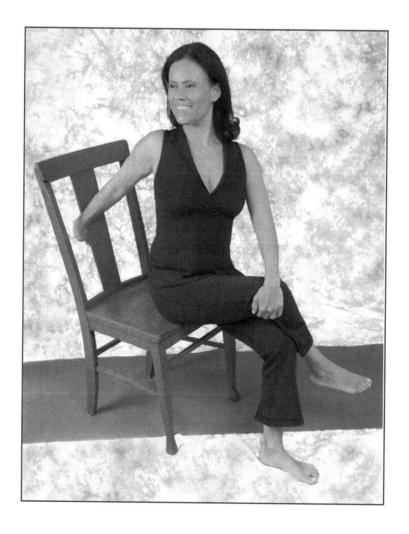

3. Inhale, straighten the spine, and then exhale, twisting gently until you feel a mild stretch in your right hip muscles and back muscles.

WHAT TO WATCH OUT FOR:

1. Avoid overtwisting and straining the back muscles.

2. Make sure you do not slouch and compress the spinal column while twisting. You have to stay tall and straight as you do this exercise.

3. Avoid pulling the knee across the body too vigorously.

BENEFITS:

1. Increases nourishment to the roots of the spinal nerves and the sympathetic nervous system.

2. Improves flexibility throughout the spinal column and also helps to mobilize the vertebrae.

3. Cleanses the body. Do it the day after overindulging with food and drink.

Seated Thigh Release

WHAT TO DO:

1. Sit at the edge of your seat in good posture, with your back straight and chin tucked.

2. Gently widen your legs until a stretch is felt in the inner thigh muscles.

3. For a deeper stretch, place hands on inner thigh muscles and press them gently outwards.

WHAT TO WATCH OUT FOR:

1. Avoid poor postural alignment and rounding of the lower back.

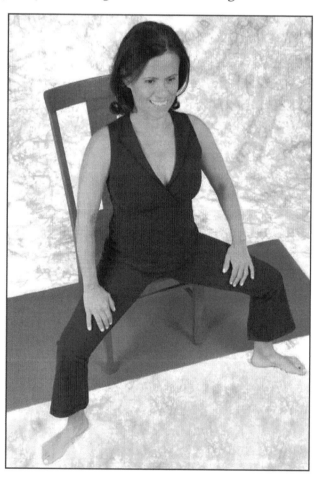

2. Do not apply too much pressure on the thighs as this can cause micro-tears in the inner thigh muscles.

BENEFITS:

1. Increases flexibility of the inner thigh, also called adductor muscles.

2. Helps to decrease trigger points in the inner thigh muscles which are quite common in women with pelvic pain.

3. Indirectly stretches out the perineum and brings blood flow to the area which is often blocked after hours of sitting.

Seated Chest Opener

WHAT TO DO:

1. Sit with good posture on the edge of your seat.

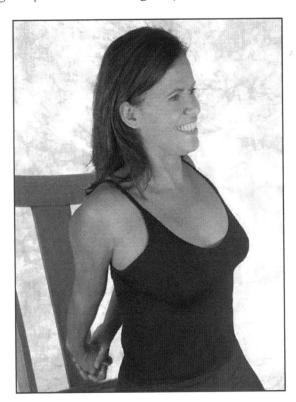

2. Clasp your hands behind your back, interlocking your fingers.

3. Roll your shoulders down and back, stretching your chest upward.

4. Raise your arms slightly upward, tucking your chin under.

WHAT TO WATCH OUT FOR:

1. Don't stick out your chin as this puts pressure on your neck.

2. Don't slouch in this pose. Sit up straight.

BENEFITS:

1. Improves posture.

2. Decreases upper and lower back pain.

3. Psychologically opens you up and puts you in a position of confidence.

Seated Reverse Kegels (Read Chapter 4 for more details)
WHAT TO DO:

1. Sit with good posture on the front of your chair with your weight evenly distributed on your sit bones.

2. Place your right hand on your right sit bone, your left hand on left sit bone, with palms facing up.

3. With your mind's eye and Tension Releasing Breath (TRB), direct your inhalation breath to your PFMs for 5 seconds, while simultaneously visualizing that your sit bones are moving apart and your pelvic floor muscles are releasing and dropping into the chair.

4. This is a very difficult exercise to do. As you get better at releasing the tension in your PFMs, you will no longer have to place your hands on your sit bones. You will be able to let go of tension in your pelvic floor in any position and at any time.

WHAT TO WATCH OUT FOR:

Avoid holding the breath and pushing out the PFMs.

BENEFITS:

Releases tension and creates flexibility in the PFMs.

Seated Diaphragmatic Breathing

WHAT TO DO:

1. Sit with good posture and place one hand on your chest and the other over your belly button.

2. Focus on your breathing. Breathe in deeply, expanding the belly outward and keeping the chest from moving too much. Then exhale with pursed lips to control the release of air, trying to keep the inhale and the exhale at the same number of seconds.

3. When you inhale, think of the word *stress* and when you exhale, think of the word *free*.

4. Focus on releasing your PFMs while doing this technique.

WHAT TO WATCH OUT FOR:

1. Do not allow thoughts besides the words *stress* and *free* to enter your mind. If this occurs, say the word *thinking* and return to the words *stress* and *free*.

2. Avoid taking in too much air at once or holding your breath. Keep your breathing smooth.

3. Don't breathe with excessive chest and neck movements, which is the opposite of diaphragmatic breathing. Non-diaphragmatic breathing is ineffective in relieving stress and clearing the mind.

BENEFITS:

1. Reduces stress and anxiety. Women with stressful jobs or those experiencing flare-ups will benefit from practicing diaphragmatic breathing at work for 10 to 20 breaths every hour on the hour.

2. Helps with pain control.

3. Allows more oxygen to enter the lungs.

4. Facilitates healing by increasing proper diaphragmatic movement and excursion of the ribs. It's important to remember that the major vessels that bring blood to the pelvic and abdominal areas travel through the diaphragm. So if the diaphragm is not moving properly, blood flow is compromised to the pelvic and abdominal organs and muscles.

We have covered a lot of ground already, laying out the key concepts for our foundation, strengthening with Kegels, stretching, and what to do at work. Now let's add the final component to our foundation, which is the foam roller series, so we can learn to release muscle pain and trigger points before they become a chronic problem.

Chapter Eight

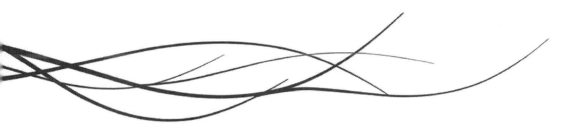

*"Always bear in mind that
your own resolution to succeed is
more important than any other thing."*
—Abraham Lincoln

Chapter 8

FOAM ROLLER MYOFASCIAL-MASSAGE AND RELEASE TECHNIQUES

Myofascial pain is a phrase that many of us are hearing more about today. Myofascial pain can be described as pain, trigger points or spasms, or sensitive areas found between muscles and fascia. Everyone knows what muscles are but fascia is a little bit more esoteric. Imagine the human body without muscles, bones, blood and fat. What would be left is a skeletal form that looks like a human body but is made of connective tissue. Fascia is a complex network of connective tissue that surrounds everything in the human body.

Many of the women I treat who suffer from pelvic conditions have moderate to severe myofascial restrictions in the muscles that attach to the pelvis and to the pelvic floor muscles. These restrictions can be classified as spasms, adhesions, knots and painful trigger points. To release these restricted muscular areas I teach all my patients to use my foam roller release series which I have included in this book.

With a foam roller you can give yourself a deep tissue massage without the hefty price tag. It's probably not as effective as a hands-on massage; however, you can do your foam rolling anywhere, anytime, and with practice your body will feel less painful, longer, softer and more flexible.

The foam roller works via the Golgi Tendon Organ (GTO) found in the area where muscles and tendon are. The GTO responds to changes in muscular tension. When you increase the pressure and/or tension in the muscles to the point where the muscle is overstrained, the GTO responds by relaxing the muscle. This is called autogenic inhibition. By exciting the GTO, muscles and fascia surrounding the muscles are able to relax helping to increase flexibility and range of motion and decreasing pain naturally.

The foam roller massage is one of my favorite self-treatment tools that uses your own body weight to release myofascial pain and trigger points found in muscles. The foam roller is tube-shaped Styrofoam that varies in shape, density and hardness. It's an inexpensive piece of equipment that is a necessary tool for women to combat conditions that afflict the pelvic floor. As you roll over your muscles, you release fascial restrictions as well as muscular trigger points and muscle spasms which restrict blood flow and do not allow your body to get rid of toxins. The foam roller also helps to soften scar tissue and muscular adhesions below surgical sites.

Many of the women I treat love their foam roller exercises and tell me they feel their muscles become softer, their pain decrease and their stress diminish. The object is to find the restrictions in muscles which tend to be hard, painful areas and to roll the painful areas slowly and deliberately for a minimum of 2 minutes until the pain decreases by at least 50 percent. Once you find a painful spot, you can also rock over the areas from side to side to increase the release of the muscle. Use the foam roller as a tool to get to know your body. You will be amazed at how many areas you will find in parts of your body that you have not thought about before. Before getting started, please read through the following charts which highlight the benefits, precautions and recommendations to consider before undertaking the foam roller series.

Table 8.1: What to Watch Out for While Performing the Foam Rolling Series

PRECAUTION
1. Avoid rolling over bony areas.
2. Avoid rolling over open wounds.
3. Avoid rolling over young, acute injuries.
4. Avoid rolling over abdominal scar younger than 6 weeks unless you get clearance from your surgeon.
5. Expect to have some muscle soreness after the rolling. If you have excessive soreness, wait 24 to 36 hours before rolling that body part again.
6. If you have circulatory problems, discuss with your doctor before starting the foam rolling exercises.
7. Avoid rolling over the abdominal area if you are experiencing moderate to severe menstrual cramps.

Table 8.2: Benefits of Self -Myofascial and Trigger Point Release with Foam Rollers

BENEFIT
1. Helps to maintain normal muscle length.
2. Improves muscle flexibility.
3. Decreases lactic acid build-up.
4. Decreases muscles adhesions and reduces scar tissue.
5. Helps eliminate trigger points, spasms and painful knots.
6. Helps increase muscle range of motion.
7. Helps to correct muscular imbalances.
8. Decreases excessive tone of muscles creating suppleness in the muscles.
9. Helps improve blood flow to muscles.
10. Releases toxins from muscles.
11. Helps reduce stress and anxiety in the body and mind.

Table 8.3: Foam Rolling Myofascial and Trigger Point Release Series

FOAM ROLLER POSITION
1. Foam Roller Upper Back Release
2. Foam Roller Sacral Rolling
3. Foam Roller Lower Back Rolling
4. Foam Roller Rolling Front of Thighs
5. Foam Roller Inner Thigh/Groin
6. Foam Roller Piriformis and Gluteal Muscle Release
7. Foam Roller Side Hip Roll - Iliotibial Band (ITB)
8. Foam Roller Quadratus Lumborum (QL) Release
9. Foam Roller Goddess
10. Foam Roller Abdominal Muscle and Scar Rolling
11.Foam Roller Sacrotuberus-Upper Hamstring

Table 8.4: Foam Rolling Recommendations

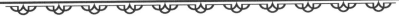

GUIDELINE
1. Drink plenty of fluids after your foam rolling sessions.
2. Roll each muscle for 1 to 3 minutes or as tolerated.
3. Keep your back straight when necessary and avoid sagging the lower back to avoid injury.
4. When rolling over painful areas or muscular knots and trigger points, roll more slowly and with shorter rolls over the painful area until you feel a muscular release or the pain starts to diminish by 50 percent. This reduction in pain may take longer than 2 minutes.
5. In addition to rolling along the body part, remember to also rock back and forth sideways with short strokes to get deeper into the trigger points and spasms you uncover.
6. For painful trigger points, keep the pressure for at least 90 seconds. Repeat as necessary until the pain decreases by 50 percent or more.
7. To reduce the effects of gravity on the body, reduce pressure and decrease pain over a muscle, do one of the following: • Keep both legs on the foam roller. • Avoid stacking the legs over each other. • Support your body as much as possible by keeping hands, feet and elbows on the floor.
8. Avoid sagging into the shoulder joint when rolling on hands. Shoulders have to be away from the ears and chest should be lifted.
9. Breathe diaphragmatically and also use Tension Releasing Breathing or TRB (see chapter 6, page 102) while rolling. Do not hold your breath while performing foam roller exercises.
10. Pay close attention to your pelvic floor muscles. Keep them relaxed as you roll over them.
11. Focus on the problem areas first until you get relief. Foam rolling can be performed everyday.

Foam Rolling Myofascial and Trigger Point Release Series
Foam Roller Upper Back Release
WHAT TO DO:

1. Place foam roller on your mid-back with your hands behind your head.

2. For neck support, keep your knees bent with your feet close to the buttocks.

3. Gently roll up and down on the thoracic spine and mid-back muscles.

4. Avoid pulling and/or hyperextending your neck.

5. Roll 1 to 2 minutes over your mid-back muscles. Focus on the painful spots and concentrate the rolling and rocking on those areas that cause you the most pain.

6. For trigger points, stay on the spots, applying consistent pressure over them for 90 seconds.

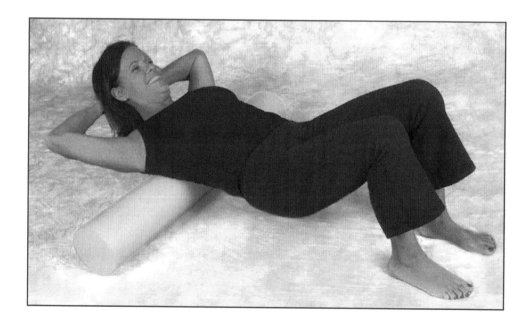

7. For muscle spasms, apply consistent pressure and do little clockwise or counterclockwise circles until pain subsides.

Foam Roller Sacral Rolling

WHAT TO DO:

1. Balance on the foam roller with both hands behind you on the floor, placing your sacrum on the foam roller.

2. Keep your hands close to the foam roller to avoid straining your shoulders.

3. Without collapsing your shoulders, gently roll up and down on the sacrum. Remember to maintain good upright posture with the chest lifted.

4. Roll 1 to 2 minutes over your sacrum. Focus on the painful spots and concentrate the rolling and rocking on that area.

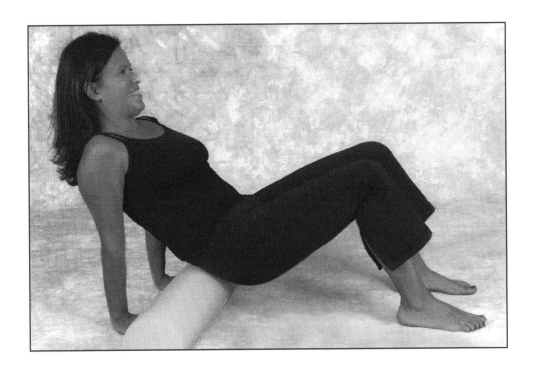

Foam Roller Lower Back Rolling

WHAT TO DO:

1. Place the foam roller on your lower back and balance on your hands behind you. Keep your hands close to the foam roller to avoid straining your shoulders.

2. Without collapsing the chest and shoulders, gently roll up and down the lower back muscles. Remember to maintain good upright posture with the chest lifted.

3. Roll 1 to 2 minutes over your lower back muscles. Focus on the painful spots and concentrate the rolling and rocking on that area.

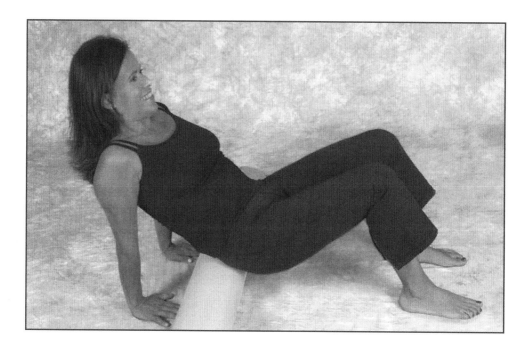

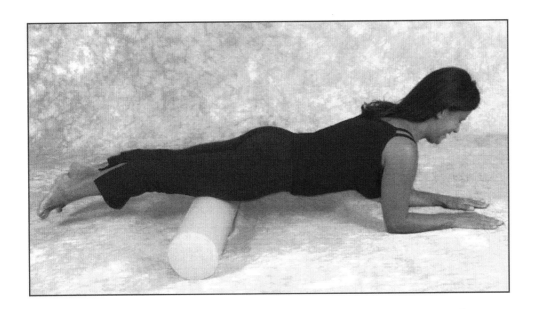

Foam Roller Rolling Front of Thighs

WHAT TO DO:

1. Balance on your elbows and place the foam roller on the front of your thighs. Keeping your abdominals slightly engaged and your back straight, roll from the upper knee to the top of the thighs. Avoid going over the kneecaps.

2. Roll 1 to 2 minutes over your thighs. Focus on the painful spots and concentrate the rolling and rocking on the areas where you find pain and restrictions.

Foam Roller Inner Thigh/Groin

WHAT TO DO:

1. Balance on your elbows and place the foam roller on the right inner thigh by flexing the right hip to the side and bending the knee. You may have to move your hands for better rolling. Your elbows should both be on one side of the roller.

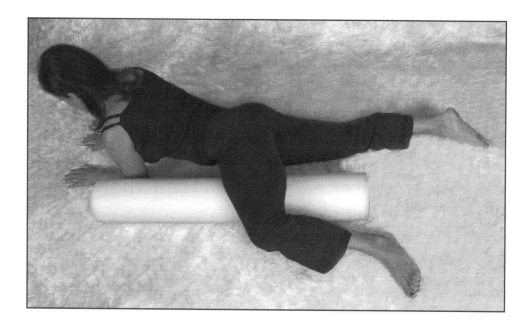

2. Slowly roll from the top of the groin to the knee.

3. Break up the rolling into the upper groin, the middle inner thigh and the lower thigh area for better emphasis. Avoid rolling over the knee joint.

4. Roll 1 to 2 minutes over your inner thighs. Focus on the painful spots and concentrate the rolling and rocking on the areas where you find pain and restrictions.

5. Switch legs and repeat on the other side.

Foam Roller Piriformis and Gluteal Muscle Release

WHAT TO DO:

1. Place the foam roller on the right buttock cheek with the ankle of the left foot across your right thigh.

2. Balancing on the right hand and right foot, slowly roll the gluteal and piriformis muscles from top to bottom. Keep your left arm balanced on the left knee.

3. Avoid collapsing the shoulders.

4. Roll 1 to 2 minutes over your gluteal and piriformis muscles. Focus on the painful spots and concentrate the rolling on that area.

5. Repeat on the other leg.

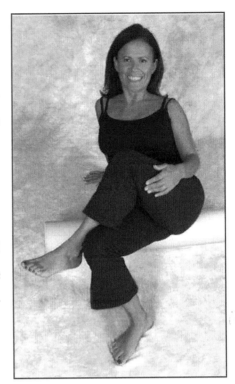

Foam Roller Side Hip Roll – Iliotibial Band (ITB)

WHAT TO DO:

1. Place the foam roller at the top of the hip bone and balance on your elbows as shown in the photo. You can also balance on the right hand if you have difficulty balancing on your elbow.

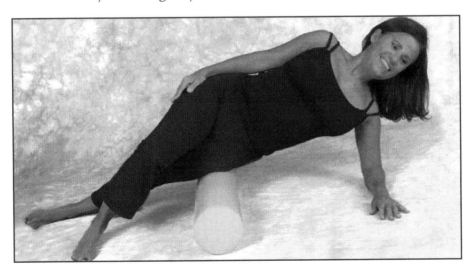

2. Keeping the body perpendicular to the foam roller, slowly roll up and down the side of the hip. Focus on the hot spots or painful spots as you roll up and down.

3. Roll 1 to 2 minutes over your ITB. Focus on the painful spots and concentrate the rolling on that area. If too painful to roll the full length of the ITB, break up the rolling into upper ITB, middle ITB, and lower ITB.

Foam Roller Quadratus Lumborum (QL) Release
WHAT TO DO:

1. Place the foam roller on the right side of the body between the rib and hip bone.

2. Balance on your right elbow and your right foot and bend your right leg in front of you.

3. Make sure you do not roll over your ribs with this exercise as you could actually break a bone if you roll over your ribs.

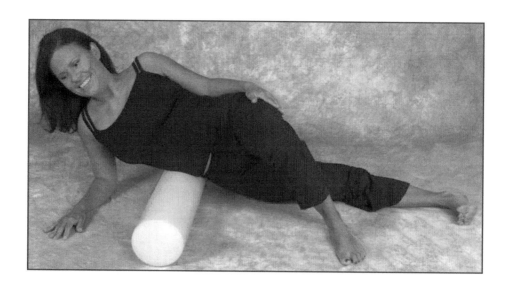

4. Roll 1 to 2 minutes over your quadratus lumborum (QL) muscles. Focus on the painful spots and concentrate the rolling on that area.

Foam Roller Goddess

WHAT TO DO:

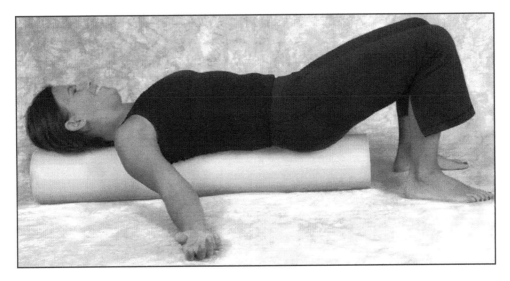

1. Lie on the foam roller with outstretched hands. Make sure to keep your entire spine on the foam roller as you practice your diaphragmatic breathing.

2. Visualize the stress leaving your body as you focus on areas of the spine that feel tight.

3. Practice your diaphragmatic breathing or mind-body techniques for 5 minutes or longer.

Foam Roller Abdominal Muscle and Scar Rolling

WHAT TO DO:

1. Balance on your elbows and place the foam roller on the abdominals. Roll from the bottom of the abdominals to the top. If you have abdominal scars, do abdominal rolls on it to release any fascial restrictions.

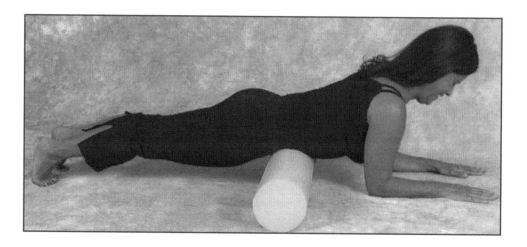

Foam Roller Sacrotuberous-Upper Hamstring

WHAT TO DO:

1. Sit high on your sit bones with legs in front of you. Make sure to maintain good, straight posture. Keeping your abdominals slightly engaged, roll gently back and forth on your sit bones.

2. Roll from the top of the sit bones to the top of the hamstring insertion, or upper back of the thighs. Focus on the hot spots and do small rolls. Be sure to avoid slumping the lower back.

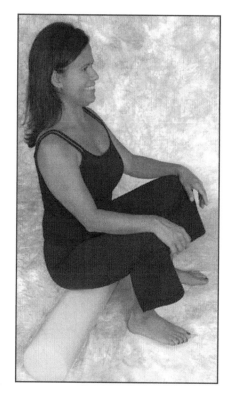

Now that our foundation is set, let's build a second layer on top in which we will directly access our own pelvic floor muscles with internal and external techniques. One of the most important aspects of your self-healing journey is to work directly on your pelvic floor muscles (PFMs). How do you do this? By accessing the muscles directly, through a variety of internal and external techniques that are outlined in Part III. Remember, think of your PFM spasms and trigger points as similar to those that some people get in their shoulders and neck muscles. Your pelvic floor muscles, like any other muscles, are susceptible to the same kinds of injuries. They can be treated in the same way we treat other body spasms, with myofascial and trigger point release, scar adhesion release, massage, and stretching.

If you approach your pelvic floor muscle or scar pain like any other muscle pain in your body, you can quickly get over your fears of doing the detective work in these sensitive areas and find the painful spots in your body. You must scientifically construct your internal and external release series with the tools in this section of the book.

Unlike the yoga, Pilates ball, and foam roller series, there is no set order for these techniques. I have laid out a toolbox for you to try, based on the tried and true techniques that I teach my patients to incorporate into their daily routines. If you find yourself hitting roadblocks or not making progress, consider seeking the help of a physical therapist that specializes in PFM work to get you on the right track. Also make sure to read the precautions in each chapter of Part III before starting your PFM release or scar program. If you are suffering from any of the symptoms listed, consult your medical doctor before you begin these techniques.

Most importantly, you must listen to what your body is saying. I firmly believe that everyone holds the key to her own healing, which is why I have written this book. Some of the techniques may elicit more pain in the short term but end up being very effective over time. When used in combination with your Kegel, breathing, yoga stretching, and Pilates ball strengthening programs, these powerful techniques can supercharge your pain relief.

Remember to use the pain mapping recommendations from Chapter 3 to really get a good sense of your body's trigger points and spasms. With a bit of grit and determination you can begin to get on the right path to reducing your painful symptoms. I cannot stress enough that you may experience an increase of your symptoms for 24 to 72 hours after you do your internal work. This is normal. Just rest, continue your reverse Kegel and stretching techniques, and resume the internal work once you feel better. The techniques in the next chapters of this book are designed to decrease hypertonicity, improve mobility, decrease pain, eliminate trigger points and improve everyday function.

In Their Own Words – Doctor to Doctor without Answers

"I had been suffering with pelvic pain for 4 months before I started physical therapy. I had been to a handful of doctors, most of whom were baffled by my condition. I had never had pelvic pain before - one day I just woke up with terrible itching and burning, and sex had become incredibly painful. I arrived at physical therapy with little hope of recovery - I had basically resigned myself to a lifetime of painful sex and discomfort (it was a regular occurrence for me to shed a few tears during my first few weeks of therapy). However, once I started a regimen (and started thinking positively), I began to see results and experience some relief. It took dedication and perseverence - physical therapy can be time consuming and sometimes painful, but I continued on day after day with the hope that one day my pain would go away. It has been about a year since the onset of my pelvic pain, and I am now almost completely pain and itch free. I have even been able to wean myself off of the medications I was on (which my doctor had prescribed to help with pelvic muscle spasms), which I never thought possible. Before the onset of my condition, I had never heard of physical therapy for pelvic pain, but I am so lucky and grateful to have found people like the therapists at Renew PT who understood my condition and helped me to recover."

Part 3
Self-Care Techniques for the Pelvic Floor

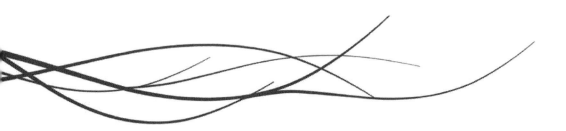

*"I have lived a long life and had many troubles,
most of which never happened."*

— *Mark Twain*

Chapter 9

DECREASING PELVIC FLOOR MUSCLE PAIN WITH INTERNAL DILATOR STRETCHES AND INTERNAL HANDS-ON TECHNIQUES

The internal techniques listed in this chapter are designed to be done with dilators or your fingers. Sometimes you may find it difficult to reach certain muscles with your fingers and will have to use your dilators. If you find yourself feeling uneasy about using dilators in general, give it some time and start slowly. With practice, you will reap the benefits of these powerful techniques.

Table 9.1: Precautions to Consider Before Starting Internal Hands-On Techniques

Get clearance from your doctor before starting vaginal or abdominal techniques outlined in this chapter, IF YOU:
1. Have just had surgery.
2. Have just given birth and have a scar from an episiotomy, perineal tear or perineal repair.
3. Have a vaginal or abdominal scar infection or bleeding.
4. Have just given birth. Wait six weeks before massaging perineal scars and only if you get clearance from your doctor.
5. Experience any increase in scar pain. Get checked to make sure the scar is healing well.
If you have started on the techniques but experience any of the following, STOP:
1. If you feel tingling down the leg or in the perineum. Stop and get off the spot as you are probably on a nerve.

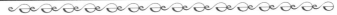

2. If you feel numbness down the leg or in the perineum. Stop and get off the spot as you are probably on an artery.
3. If you smell a foul odor coming from your vagina, abdominal or perineal scar. This could be a sign of infection and must be reported to your caregiver.
4. If you get on a spot that has a pulse. You are probably on an artery and want to avoid compressing into the blood supply.
General Guidelines:
1. Avoid massaging and pressing the tendinous arch of the levator ani muscles. This tendon feels like a cooked spaghetti noodle and is usually very painful to touch. See Diagram 3.1 on page 35 for the location of this tendon.
2. You may be able to massage more vigorously if you have had an internal Botox injection to relax your PFMs.

Dilators

A great way to eliminate painful trigger points and to get your PFMs supple and pain-free again is to do daily dilator stretches. At first many of my patients

feel strange about doing this kind of exercise, in such a personal area, with a thing that looks like a small dildo. Many of you will also have fear and anxiety having to look at and touch your vaginas. Just as you would stretch your hamstrings on a daily basis, stretching your vaginal muscles is a normal and necessary thing to do if you are suffering from conditions 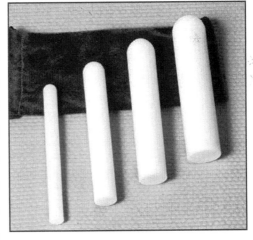 like painful sex or muscle spasms. Look at stretching your vaginal muscles with a dilator not in a sexual context but as a medical necessity that will help you regain a pain-free life. For many of you, you will not achieve pain-free sex unless you incorporate intravaginal stretching on a daily basis into your exercise program. This type of therapy is an integral part of your sexual healing.

Dilators are healing devices that will assist you in stretching out your PFMs and reducing pain associated with sex and activities of daily living. Many women have pain during intercourse, and the dilator is a great tool that helps open up and release this area. Dilators are also great for relieving deep trigger points found in the inner layers of the PFMs.

Dilators come in different graduated sizes. Most of my patients start with extra small and gradually move up as their muscles become stretched, less painful, and open. These different sizes help to stretch the vaginal muscles so that sexual penetration is not painful. Some of my patients who had experienced intense pain with penetration but who have now graduated to the largest dilator, still fear having sexual relations even

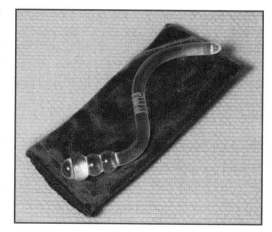

Crystal Wand

though their muscles are stretched out and pain-free. With practice, dilators can help you overcome your fear of penetration.

Another tool that is a great resource is called the Crystal Wand. This curved device can be used for hard to reach spots in the innermost layers of the pelvic floor.

To reduce any anxiety you might have before starting the PFM stretching, become familiar with your dilator before your session. Feel the dilator's hard smooth texture, press it against your body and examine the different sizes in your set, if you already have more than one. Another great way to prepare yourself for this type of stretching is to meditate for 5 to 10 minutes before you begin your session, incorporating diaphragmatic breathing to release tension and reduce anxiety. I find that many of my patients also try to see the humor in their situation and find that giving the dilator a name keeps the internal work lighter and less emotionally charged.

Dilator sizes vary in their diameter, getting progressively wider. Some dilator sets come with 4 different sizes, and others up to 8. The set that I use with my patients has 4 dilators to a set, and I number them 1 to 4, from smallest to largest (see photo on page 161). To use them correctly, make sure you have a basic knowledge of your vaginal anatomy and muscles as I have defined in Chapter 3 of the book. I also find that when my patients are consistent with their exercises they experience less pain with sex, sitting, positional changes and standing, and are ultimately happier.

In Their Own Words – One Patient's Pre- and Post-Surgical Story

"I noticed the first symptoms of vestibulodynia (VVS) about six months after my wedding. For a while, I had been treated with strong antibiotics for a persistent stomach parasite, and each of the 3 courses of antibiotics had left me with bad yeast infections. These yeast infections never seemed to go away even though I eventually found a doctor who gave me daily oral antifungals. During this time, I avoided sex because sex with a yeast infection is a pretty bad idea. It hurts and you can pass it back and forth between partners. Even when I finally tested negative for yeast, the pain was still there. In fact, it was more intense than before. On penetration, I felt a tearing, burning sensation that temporarily disappeared but returned more intensely after sex. It felt like I was on fire, it was unbearable. For as long as 48 hours after sex, I was plagued by burning, itching and stabbing sensations in my vestibular area. It felt like having a UTI each time I had sex.

"My doctor said she believed it was vestibulodynia and suggested I try a steroid cream. In Australia (where I was living at that time), they tend to be more conservative in their medical approach. While this is often a good thing, I think a more aggressive treatment at the outset yields a better outcome for vestibulodynia. Steroid cream was commonly prescribed 5 years ago, but it is rarely done today because it has been known to further weaken the skin of the vulva, making it even more prone to tearing. After a few months she referred me to a gynecologist, who was very kind and understanding. She put me back on daily oral antifungals and prescribed physical therapy. I had 2 sessions with the therapists before being discharged, but I did not get any better. I tried a low-oxalate diet, which did nothing but make me skeletally thin. Then I saw an acupuncturist who may have helped my sinuses, but did nothing for my VVS.

"In 2004, I moved back to New York and decided to consult a pioneering doctor in Boston who was amazing. She listened to my history and treated the condition very aggressively. Over the course of the next 2 years, I had some improvement, mostly from lidocaine cream. Unfortunately, I just didn't respond well enough and it became clear that I would be one of the very rare cases for whom surgery was going to be the best option. In 2006, my doctor referred me to Isa Herrera at Renew PT to begin physical therapy in preparation for my surgery. I had a very dim view of physical therapy based on my experiences in Sydney. But Isa proved to be my secret weapon against VVS. She has made it her life's work to understand how to unlock the body to lessen the grip of vaginal pain. Isa got me ready both physically and psychologically to face the frightening realities of a vestibulectomy. Whenever I would get discouraged, she would help me build up my mental framework and shore me up against the frustrations of this very mentally-challenging disease.

"I would like to use this space to talk a little about the surgery itself. I don't think doctors are entirely clear about how big an impact this surgery has on your body and mind. Maybe they don't want you to build it up and be afraid or maybe they just don't get it. But I feel that having all the information at hand would have been better, so I will relate my experience here.

"A vestibulectomy is not a small surgery. It is not a 'glorified episiotomy' as I have heard it called. The surgery I had, which in all fairness was more radical than average, was brutal. I bled far longer than the aftercare sheet said I would. I was unable to leave Boston after the surgery because my bleeding was so heavy the doctor wanted me to stay near the hospital to be on the safe side. I was in ridiculously searing pain for the first ten days or so. And even once the nightmare was over, there was the plain fact that I was physically too small for even a routine pap smear with a speculum. Isa helped me stretch out the vaginal opening with dilators, which are basically just medical-grade dildos, over the course of a long, long time. My recovery period from surgery to pain-free sex took 8 months. But then again, you may have caught that last bit: pain-free sex. Yes, the surgery is horrible and the recovery is only slightly less so, but I am 95 percent better. No more burning and itching after sex. Next month will mark one year since the surgery and thanks to my doctor in Boston and the fantastic care at Renew PT, I can wear tight jeans, ride a bike, and have sex like a newlywed."

Getting Started

To start, you should have a mirror, pillows, vaginal lubricant, and if you like, non-latex gloves. For vaginal lubricants I like to use FireFly™, Slippery Wet™ or old-fashioned olive oil, vitamin E oil, or rose oil. Make sure you do not have allergies to any of these products. I am also a big fan of lubricants that are organic and alcohol free, if you have access to any of these products. For organic and hypoallergenic products, visit your local health food store or your local sex shop.

The vaginal stretching exercises can be done in several different positions, but to familiarize yourself with the techniques, starting off in a semi-reclined position with a pillow under your head will work great. If your hip muscles are very tight or if you become uncomfortable, place a pillow under each thigh so that your knees are supported. Later on you can experiment with one leg up supported on the toilet or bench. You can even try lying on your side, which is also a great position.

Table 9.2: Internal Techniques for Pelvic Muscle Release Using a Dilator or Finger

NAME OF TECHNIQUE
1. General Pelvic Floor Muscle Stretching
2. Pelvic Floor Muscle Clock Stretching
3. Pelvic Floor Myofascial Release
4. Internal PFM Trigger Point Release
5. Internal PFM Cross Friction Fiber Massage
6. Internal PFM Half-Moon Strumming Massage

General Pelvic Floor Muscle Stretching

WHAT TO DO:

1. Clean your dilator with hot water and soap. Avoid using antibacterial wipes and antibacterial soaps. Use the same soap that you use to clean your body. I recommend hypoallergenic soap like Aveeno™. Some silicone dilators can be cleaned by placing them in boiling water for a few minutes.

2. To keep the dilator warm, place it in a cup of warm water until you are ready to use it.

3. Apply a generous amount of lubricant to your vaginal opening. Dry off the dilator and place plenty of lubricant on its tip.

4. Practice diaphragmatic breathing for a couple of breaths and do a couple of reverse Kegels or contract/relax Kegels as defined in Part II. This will help relax your PFM before insertion of the dilator, and will make your experience more comfortable. You may also want to do your yoga series before you begin so you can be in a more relaxed state.

5. When you are ready both mentally and physically, slowly insert the dilator into your vaginal opening, angling the dilator downwards towards your tailbone. The dilators are usually 6 to 8 inches long but initially try inserting it 2 to 3 inches. ONLY insert the dilator to your physical and emotional comfort level. The dilator is not meant to go all the way inside; you should be able to hold on to the end of it. Continue inserting it, stopping periodically to practice your diaphragmatic breathing, your reverse Kegel, and your contract/relax Kegels, which will help you insert it deeper.

6. Avoid inserting or pressing the dilator in the 12 o'clock or top position because your bladder is located there and there are no muscles to stretch at this position. Inserting it in this position could also cause bladder pain, or worse, could possibly damage the bladder tissue.

7. At first keep the dilator inside the vagina anywhere from 5 minutes to an hour everyday, depending on how much you can tolerate. When you feel you are ready, you can thrust the dilator in and out to simulate sexual intercourse. Do not do more than you can tolerate. This in-and-out motion can be done at any time during your dilator routine and with any size dilator. The key thing is to make sure you are psychologically and emotionally prepared to do it.

8. Try advancing to the next size dilator after a week or 2 of consistent exercising with the smaller dilator. Do not advance to the next size unless you are comfortable with inserting it, moving it around, and there is little or no pain when using your current dilator.

9. To advance to the next dilator it is sometimes helpful to switch back and forth between dilator sizes for comfort and to get used to the larger size. When you switch between sizes, relubricate and insert slowly especially if going from smaller to bigger. Remember that you will decide how to advance your own dilator stretching program. The key concept to ensure success and to put you on the road to pain-free sex is being consistent with your dilator exercises. If you fall off the wagon with your exercises, start your program again as soon as possible. Remember to always be gentle with yourself and do not let your mind fill with negative self-talk. Be gentle with yourself as you progress because it takes time!

10. Your goal is to be able to fit a dilator comfortably inside your vagina that is one size bigger than your partner's penis.

Pelvic Floor Muscle Clock Stretching

GETTING STARTED:

The pelvic floor muscle clock stretching techniques work great for women who are having trouble getting the dilators into their vaginas, or for those women who have pain with initial penetration, painful scars, or spasms in their muscles. For this method, imagine again that your vaginal opening is a clock.

To review, 12 o'clock is by the clitoris, 6 o'clock is by the rectum, 3 o'clock is to the left and 9 o'clock is to the right. Using your smallest dilator or finger, start stretching your vagina using the clock as visualization. Remember that the PFMs are divided into 3 layers, each layer corresponding to the knuckles of the finger and progressively deeper inside the vagina. The first PFM layer is knuckle 1, the second PFM layer is knuckle 2, and the third PFM layer is knuckle 3.

Diagram 9.1: Clock

WHAT TO DO:

1. Focus your stretching from 3 to 9 o'clock positions avoiding 12 o'clock where the bladder is located.

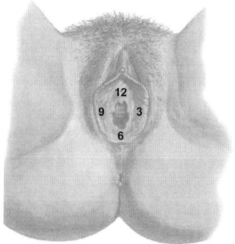

2. Start with PFM Layer 1, then progress to Layer 2, and then to Layer 3, only when you feel comfortable and confident.

3. Press around the clock for 30

Base Image: Netter Images

to 60 seconds or until you feel a release in the vaginal muscles. You can go around the clock 2 to 3 times or you can stay on the same spot for 3 repetitions of 30 to 60 seconds.

4. For women who have just had babies or for those who have undergone surgeries, it is best to wait at least 6 weeks and get cleared by your childbirth caregiver before starting your clock stretching program.

5. The main thing is to decrease the pain as you press into the muscles. I always aim for at least 50 percent reduction in pain when I do the clock stretches on my patients.

6. Oils that can be used for stretching are vitamin E oil, rose oil and any lubricant that is organic and alcohol free.

Pelvic Floor Muscle Myofascial Release

GETTING STARTED:

Myofascial stretching and release of the PFMs is one of the best techniques in this chapter to improve mobility, decrease pain, increase strength, and decrease hypertonicity, creating more supple muscles. To visualize the technique, imagine that your PFMs are 3-dimensional, like a tube. There are 3 layers to the tube from superficial to the deepest layer. The tube is further divided with 2 outer walls on the left and right, an inferior wall, near the rectum, and a superior wall, towards the bladder. Now imagine that the walls of the tube described above are divided in half the long way, a right half and a left half. The left half corresponds to the clock at 1, 2, 3, 4, 5, 6 o'clock, and the right half corresponds to the 6, 7, 8, 9, 10, 11, and 12 o'clock position. This methodology is also helpful for doing advanced pain mapping as well as to help you track the location of your pain.

WHAT TO DO:

1. Place some lubricant on your dilator or finger and insert your finger or dilator into the third or deepest layer at the 2 o'clock position. On your finger this corresponds to the third knuckle. This technique requires that you

Diagram 9.2: Cylinder and Clock

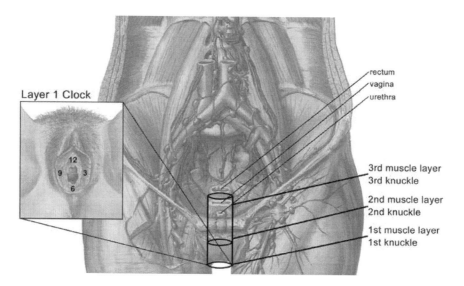

Base Image: Netter Images

apply gentle yet firm pressure throughout the PFM layer by layer.

2. Using your dilator or finger apply gentle yet firm pressure for 20 to 30 seconds on the left half of the third layer at 2 o'clock. Repeat for 3, 4, 5, and 6 o'clock positions in the third layer. Then continue on the left side and repeat the 2 to 6 o'clock positions on the second and then first PFM layers.

3. Once you have completed the left half of the myofascial technique, go to the right side and repeat the same 20 to 30 second pressure release at 10, 9, 8, 7, and 6 o'clock positions through the deepest PFM Layer 3 to the superficial PFM Layer 1.

4. You may find very painful spots as you move through the layers and around the clock. If you come across a layer that is extremely painful, you have found a trigger point. Take note of its location and use the trigger point release method that follows to attack and eliminate it.

Internal Pelvic Floor Muscle Trigger Point Release

GETTING STARTED:

Use this method hand-in-hand with the myofascial release technique. Trigger point therapy is not a quick-fix solution for chronic pelvic pain. It can take weeks and even months to stabilize the pain. The one thing that is important to understand is that once you have mastered these basic techniques you will be able to take back control over the pain. To be successful with the trigger point release techniques, you have to scientifically map your pain level and trigger point to see how the pain changes and diminishes over time. Once you increase your awareness of these areas you can also better focus your mental healing imagery as well.

WHAT TO DO:

1. For this technique, use the same PFM description as outlined in the internal pelvic floor muscle myofascial release technique from earlier in this chapter.

2. Your objective is to find the painful trigger points in the PFMs and press them for 90 seconds until you eliminate the pain or decrease the pain by 50 percent.

3. You may have to press into the trigger points for several 90-second repetitions as one might not give you the relief right away. When you press on these painful spots avoid pressing too hard and stay below a pain level of 5 out of 10 (0= no pain, 10 = worst pain you ever had).

4. Many times the trigger points you find will refer pain to another part of your body. Remember that this is quite normal. Just continue to work hard to eliminate your trigger points as described above. When I find trigger points in my patients, I find areas that either have small bumps in them or feel raised or hard.

Internal Pelvic Floor Muscle Cross Friction Fiber Massage

GETTING STARTED:

Cross friction fiber massage requires a small motion, about half an inch to an inch of back and forth movement "across the fiber" of the pelvic floor muscles in a perpendicular motion. This technique is useful in places where you find pain, scar tissue, or bumps in the muscles. The amount of pressure should be moderate and really depends on your pain tolerance. This internal massage may cause some amount of discomfort, but it should never be too painful. I would avoid going over a level 5 pain (0 = no pain, 10 = worst pain ever) when performing this massage. Avoid massaging over the tendinous arch of the levator ani muscles. It will feel like a spaghetti noodle and almost always causes pain.

WHAT TO DO:

Diagram 9.3: Cross Friction Massage

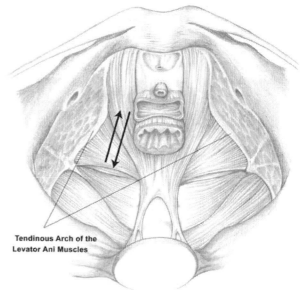

Tendinous Arch of the
Levator Ani Muscles

1. Imagine again that the PFMs are a tube divided into 2 halves, a right half and a left half. The muscle fibers of the 2 halves generally run from superior to inferior, or top to bottom, and are parallel to each other. See diagram.

2. Massage across the PFM fiber in a perpendicular motion, which will be in an internal to external, or in to out motion across the muscle fiber, as in Diagram 9.3.

Arrows represent direction of massage with dilator or finger. Try to avoid the tendinous arch of the levator ani muscles, as it will almost always elicit pain. Base image: Winston Johnson

3. Insert your lubricated dilator or finger up to the third knuckle and start to search for painful muscle spots or spots that feel like there is a knot, scar or bumps in the muscle. Once you have identified a spot, use an internal to ex-

ternal massage stroke with either your finger or the tip of the dilator directly on the painful spot or across a bigger part of the muscle. For example, use an internal to external stroke at 3 o'clock in Layer 2 on the left side. Map your pain and track your progress.

4. Perform the cross friction massage for at least 3 to 5 minutes and then move to another location in the same side, if necessary. Cross friction massage helps to break down adhesions, spasms, and scar tissue, but it does take time.

5. I recommend that you wait at least 24 hours before doing the cross friction massage again just to see how you respond to this technique.

6. Keep track of your overall pain levels as this is your best gauge as to whether this method is good for you. You may have to try it a couple of times before determining if this method is the right one to incorporate into your healing program.

Internal Pelvic Floor Muscle Half–Moon Strumming Massage

GETTING STARTED:

Strumming is another great way to help release painful knots, spasms and trigger points in the PFMs. Strumming is similar to cross friction except that the motion is parallel, and goes along the muscle fiber. It is generally less painful than cross friction. Strumming and cross friction go hand-in-hand; you can mix and match the cross friction and strumming techniques based on your own internal palpation of your pelvic floor. Once you get used to your own muscles and locations of pain and spasm, you will begin to develop an intuition towards the best combination to alleviate your condition. Be your own detective, get to know your body, and listen to what your body is telling you. Tune into the messages that your body is sending, and you will be able to have better control.

Diagram 9.4: Half-Moon Strumming

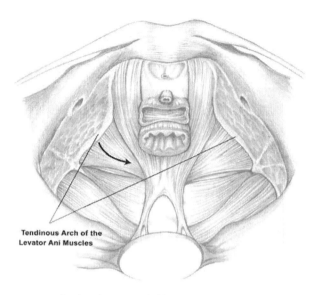

Tendinous Arch of the
Levator Ani Muscles

Arrow represent direction of massage with dilator or finger. Try to avoid the tendinous arch of the levator ani muscles, as it will almost always elicit pain. Base image: Winston Johnson

WHAT TO DO:

1. Strumming massage, as opposed to cross friction massage, is a type of massage that is performed in the direction of the pelvic floor muscle fiber. So this massage is from superior to inferior, or top to bottom.

2. First work the right half of the PFM and then work the left half, massaging layer by layer from deepest Layer 3 to superficial Layer 1. For example, strum from 3 to 4 o'clock in Layer 2 on the left side.

3. As with cross friction, always map your pain and techniques, so over time you can get a good scientific sense of what is working.

4. Avoid masaging the arcus tendon of the levator ani muscle. It feels like thick cooked spaghetti and will usually elicit pain.

Hand in hand with these internal techniques are the external massage and release strategies discussed in the next chapter.

Chapter Ten

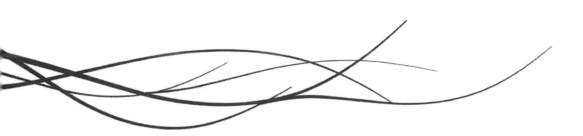

"Disciples and devotees...what are most of them doing?
Worshipping the teapot instead of drinking the tea! "
— *Wei Wu Wei*

Chapter 10

DECREASING PELVIC FLOOR MUSCLE SYMPTOMS AND PAIN WITH EXTERNAL HANDS-ON TECHNIQUES

External self-care techniques are great tools to help normalize PFMs, increase flexibility, improve range of motion and eliminate painful trigger points and spasms. I often recommend that my patients use these external tools when they are not comfortable doing intravaginal or intrarectal work or need a rest to recover from their internal PFM work. The external techniques are very effective in reducing and relieving female pelvic symptoms and are easy to do. These techniques may help you locate trigger points that could be referring pain and other symptoms to the PFMs, hip/pelvic region and contributing to leaking, urgency, sexual dysfunction, clitoral or vulvar pain. These external techniques also help smooth out the muscle fibers and connective tissue that can easily contribute in subtle ways to your PFM conditions. Also included in this chapter are strain-counterstrain and psoas release therapy. These two therapies are lifesavers for my patients and are very easy to do and to incorporate into your healing journey. This chapter also covers skin rolling for the sacrum, abdominal and inner thigh muscles. Skin rolling really gets the fascia moving and helps to normalize muscle tension and restrictions.

Please read this whole chapter carefully before doing any of these amazing self-care techniques. If you read everything first, you will get a more global picture of the task that lies ahead of you. You can then try all the techniques and focus on the ones that bring you the most pain relief. Always listen to your body when performing these techniques. Your body will signal to you when something is right or wrong. Don't override your body signals because, if you do, you risk a flare-up or more pain or more leaking. Read the guidelines below to make sure you know some of the basic principles and how not to hurt yourself. Now that you've been informed, go have fun with the work and enjoy the process. There is only one way to do this and that is to go into the rabbit hole so you can truly unwind your conditions and get those long-term results that you desire and need.

In Their Own Words - Healing My Pain Using Isa's Great Tools

"I came to Renew PT for pelvic pain syndrome called vulvodynia or vestibulitis. At Renew, I was given cold laser treatments and massages for specific muscles that were very tight or had trigger points in them. Isa also recorded my muscular tension with a machine that does biofeedback. In just over a month of twice weekly treatments, I am completely pain-free in huge part to Isa's treatment, but also from doing the homework she assigned me. I did these regularly even when I was traveling or could not make my appointments.

"Isa designed a program that included stretching, internal and external massages, and myofascial releases. What I like about Renew is that Isa approaches pelvic pain from multiple perspectives. It is not just muscular, neuropathic or stress related — she customizes a program to fit each individual person and then gives homework for empowerment. I highly recommend the excellent services and staff at Renew PT. I am here to say that I am pain-free because of their care."

General Guidelines for Working on Trigger Points

WHEN DOING THESE TECHNIQUES, WATCH OUT FOR THE FOLLOWING:

1. You may experience muscle soreness 24 to 72 hours afterward. This is normal.

2. These techniques can be very painful. When you start to touch these areas, the pain may be higher than you expected. Please stay within a pain level of three to five rating or within your pain tolerance. Pain scale measurement is as follows: Rate your pain from 0 to 10 (pain scale 0 = no pain, 10 = worst pain you ever had in your life).

3. You may see some bruising/redness on your skin after doing some of the rolling techniques. If this occurs, be gentler with the rolling, but do not become alarmed.

4. Your PFMs may respond by tightening when you first start to use these techniques. If this occurs, do the reverse Kegel exercise and couple it with diaphragmatic breathing. Performing the breath with the reverse Kegel will help calm everything down.

5. Avoid holding tension in your PFMs because you are experiencing too much pain. If your PFMs get tense or start to contract and become tight, back off and use less pressure with the tools. Listen to your body.

6. Incorporate Tension Release Breathing (TRB) as described in Chapter 6 into the techniques especially if you are experiencing pain with the external trigger points. Like diaphragmatic breathing, TRB will help to calm the pain down.

7. Stay away from pulses especially in the abdominal and hip area. Never press into a pulse.

8. Try one to two techniques at a time. If you try too many at once, you will not know what works best for you.

9. For trigger point therapy, press into the spots slowly and gently. Also release the pressure on the trigger point slowly.

10. When in doubt about how to do the external tools, don't do the technique. You don't want to hurt yourself. Instead seek the help of a trained pelvic floor physical therapist who can guide you through the process.

11. Show this book and the techniques that you want to do to your MD, caregiver and/or physical therapist first. It is best to err on the side of safety.

12. Always pay attention to your breathing. Breathe rhythmically and deeply. Avoid holding your breath. Keep your jaw relaxed.

13. Use aromatherapy oils of high quality such as those sold at *www.youngliving.com./en_US/*. To order Young Living Oils use my subscriber number #1422496 to register. The Young Living Oils that work great for these painful areas are basil, lavender and balsam fir. Read through the Young Living website and choose oils that not only reduce pain but also relax the mind. You may need to find a certified aromatherapist to help you. I also make a great oil called Pain Be Gone that works miraculously on these painful areas. Using oils for massages and trigger point therapy can help reduce pain and stress.

Table 10.1: External Techniques for Relief of Pelvic Pain and the Normalization of PFM and Female Bladder Function

NAME OF TECHNIQUE
1. Labia Stretch, Roll and Cross Friction Massage
2. Abdominal Rolling
3. Lower Back Massage
4. Sacral Rolling
5. Inner Thigh Massage, Skin Rolling and Trigger Point Release
6. External PFMs Trigger Point Therapy for Superficial Transverse Perineal Muscle, Ischiocavernosus Muscle, Bulbospongiosus, Levator Ani, and Perineal Body
7. Abdominal External Muscular Trigger Point Therapy
8. Lower Body External Muscular Trigger Point Therapy
9. Upper Body and Bone Areas External Trigger Point Therapy
10. Gluteal Muscles External Body Trigger Point Therapy
11. Strain-Counterstrain for Obturator Internus
12. Contract/Relax for Obturator Internus
13. Psoas Release
14. PNF Contract/Relax for Global PFMs Relaxation
15. Anal Rim Massage
16. Suprapubic External Bladder Trigger Points
17. Perineum Pressure Point Technique
18. Clitoral Hood Release and Stretch with Anatomy Explanation

Labia Stretch, Roll and Cross Friction Massage

GETTING STARTED:

The labia are truly amazing female structures that provide us with access to nerves, muscles, and erectile tissue. This type of stretching and mobilization is great for women who are having pain with initial penetration or for women whose pelvic floor muscles are too tight and painful for intercourse. Working on the labia will also help women suffering from pudendal nerve neuralgia. When performing these techniques, focus on increasing the flexibility and suppleness of the labial tissue. These techniques are also great to use when you have your period and do not want to do internal vaginal work.

Diagram 10.1: Labia Stretch

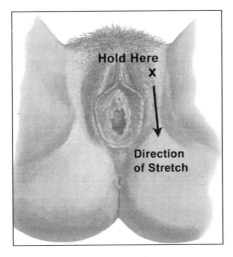

Base Image Source: Netter Images

WHAT TO DO:

Labia Stretch

Anchor your finger on the top of the right labia majora near the clitoris. Place the thumb of the opposite hand at the bottom of the same labia and stretch downward. Hold for 30 seconds to 1 minute, repeating 2 to 3 times and then switch to the other labia.

Labia Roll (no illustration)

Pinch the right labia majora between the thumb and the forefinger. Roll the tissue gently between the fingers until you reach the bottom. You can roll the labia tissue in either an upward or downward direction; choose the direction that is least painful for you. Repeat 2 to 3 times and then switch sides. Be very gentle and soft when working on this delicate structure.

Diagram 10.2 : Labia Cross Friction Massage

Direction
of Massage

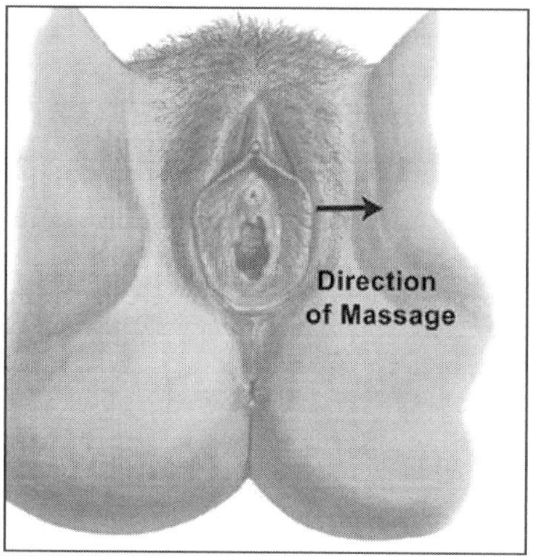

Base Image Source: Netter Images

Labia Cross Friction Massage

Place your index or forefinger on the top of your right labia majora. Gently massage the tissue across the labia from side to side until you reach the bottom. Repeat 2 to 3 times and then switch sides.

Abdominal Rolling

GETTING STARTED:

The PFMs are influenced by the fascia of the abdominal muscles. When the PFMs are painful, in spasms, and lack mobility, the abdominal muscle can sometimes respond by becoming tight, painful and developing trigger points. I find that when abdominal massage and rolling are incorporated into the treatment sessions, my patients are better able to tolerate the intravaginal stretches and massage more easily. Many of my patients tell me that after the abdominal massage they can insert their dilator or finger into their vaginas with more ease and less pain. The abdominal muscles may also have trigger points in them, and you will discover yours as you massage and explore the abdominals.

If you come across a very painful trigger point – and sometimes these painful spots can refer pain elsewhere in the pelvis – hold the spot for 90 seconds until the pain subsides. Repeat the 90-second holds until you have either eliminated the trigger point or reduced the pain by 50 percent. See upcoming paragraphs on abdominal trigger point therapy for more information.

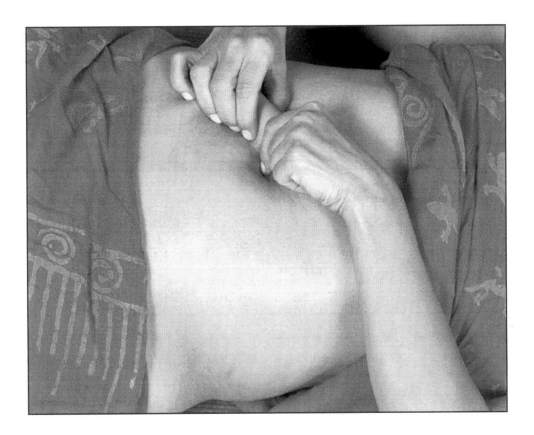

Remember that it's important to determine your pain level at the start of any treatment so that you can track your progress. To facilitate abdominal rolling, place a heating pad or hot water bottle on your tummy for ten minutes before you start rolling. The heat has to be low heat. Avoid high heat because you could burn yourself. Trust me: patients inadvertently burn themselves at home all the time. You can roll the abdominal muscles with or without an oil. First, try without an oil; if that is too painful then think about using aromatherapy and choose an oil that helps you to relax and glide over the abdominal muscle with ease and less or no pain. Look into Young Living Oils to help release pain, spasms and help with digestion. The Young Living Oils I use most frequently for the abdominals include lavender and peppermint.

Precaution for Abdominal Rolling

Your physician will provide the guidelines, but generally you must wait until six weeks after your abdominal surgery before starting these techniques. (Also check with your doctor if you are recovering from another type of surgery.) This is when the abdominal scar is almost fully healed. While your doctor may give you permission to start earlier, do not begin abdominal rolling/massage any earlier than six weeks after abdominal or laparoscopic surgery without medical clearance. During these surgeries small incisions are made into the abdomen. Also check with your MD regarding time frames for Cesarean or myomectomy surgeries.

WHAT TO DO:

1. Get a pleasant aromatherapy oil with a scent that helps you to relax as you work with your abdominal rolling. Lavender oil is a great scent and helps reduce bladder symptoms. I use Young Living Oils. You can order these at *www.youngliving.com/en_US/* and use my number #1422496 when ordering. Make sure to obtain medical clearance from your MD before using any aromatherapy oils.

2. Cup your abdominal muscles by placing index fingers near each other so they are gently touching and place your thumbs superior to the other fingers as in the photo above. Stay superficial on your abdominal muscle and avoid grabbing the muscles too deeply.

3. Gently glide your fingers toward your thumbs repeating 10 to 20 times and change your hand placement. For simplicity's sake, I have divided the abdominal muscles into an upper part and lower part. Roll the lower part first, focusing on upward motions. Make sure to cover all the lower abdominal muscles and then switch to rolling the upper abdominal muscles in a downward motion.

4. Remember to pay attention to the trigger points and handle or treat them as previously described in this chapter.

5. Finish your abdominal rolling by gently massaging your entire abdominal region with clockwise circles.

6. Try to roll your abdominals 5 to 15 minutes on a daily basis and perform at least 20 clockwise circles to end your massage.

Lower Back Massage

GETTING STARTED:

Many of the women I treat with pelvic pain also suffer from lower back pain. These two conditions go hand-in-hand. Massaging the lower back is important to help release tension and trigger points in this region.

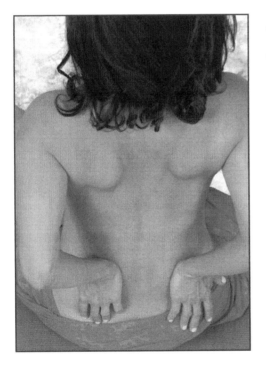

WHAT TO DO:

1. Learn to massage yourself in different positions and use firm pressure, avoiding excessive pain.

2. Massage down the lower back muscles using long downward strokes. You can use your knuckles or hands. Make sure to cover the entire lower back area.

3. Using your right hand, massage your right lower back muscles for five to ten minutes. Then switch sides massaging your left lower back muscles with your left hand.

4. For painful trigger points found in any of the back muscles, apply sustained

pressure over the painful area for 90 seconds. Repeat as necessary until the pain has decreased by at least 50 percent or the pain is totally eliminated.

5. A great addition to the low back rolling is to massage your low back outward from the spine along the line of your hip bone using your knuckles. This can be very painful at first, but continue to do this massage until the pain has diminished by 50 percent or more. The goal here is to be pain-free.

Sacral Rolling

GETTING STARTED:

The sacrum houses many of the nerve roots that innervate the abdominal organs, PFMs and hip muscles. It is critical to keep the tissues in this area free and supple. One of the great tools that I give my patients is sacral rolling.

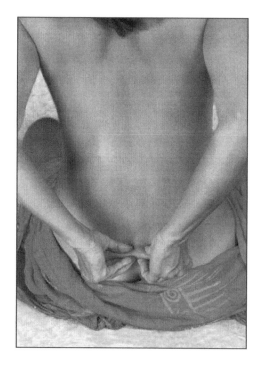

WHAT TO DO:

1. Cup the skin in your sacral area and roll it in the same manner that you would roll your abdominals. See the photo for hand placement.

2. Roll the sacrum upward for two to five minutes on a daily basis. In the beginning, sacral rolling might be painful, but over time as you roll the sacrum it will become less painful to do.

3. The goal is to be pain-free when doing the sacral rolling.

Inner Thigh Massage, Skin Rolling and Trigger Point Release

GETTING STARTED:

The inner thigh muscles require special attention because of their close proximity to the pelvis and PFMs. The inner thigh muscles can develop spasms, trigger points and adhesions in them as a response to what is happening internally in the PFMs. These tissue abnormalities can make sitting, walking and positional changes painful. The trigger points in the inner thigh can refer to the bladder and reproduce bladder symptoms such as urgency. To restore proper function, muscle length, and flexibility to the inner thigh muscles, use the three techniques described below.

Long Deep Inner Thigh Strokes

WHAT TO DO:

1. Massage the inner thigh muscles from the knee to the upper groin, using long deep strokes for five to ten minutes.

2. If performing the massage without oil is too painful, you can use a small drop of oil or massage cream to make the gliding less painful or use aromatherapy oils such as my Pain Be Gone available at *www.RenewPT.com*.

Inner Thigh Skin Rolling

WHAT TO DO:

1. Roll your inner thigh muscles from the knee to the groin using the rolling techniques described under abdominal rolling. Try not to use an oil and stay superficially on the skin so you target the inner thigh fascia.

2. Roll the inner thigh for five to ten minutes or as tolerated.

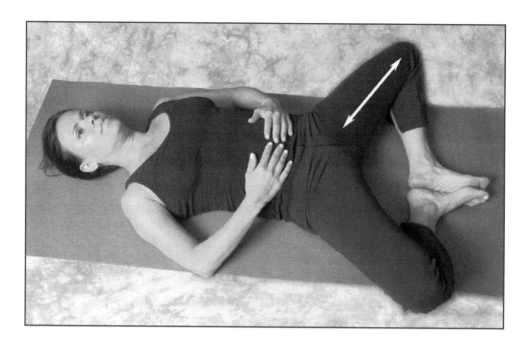

Inner Thigh Trigger Point Release

WHAT TO DO:

1. The inner thigh muscles can develop trigger points in them as a response to pelvic pain. Search for these trigger points by running your hands slowly along your inner thigh muscles. A trigger point will feel like a hard, small ball and will produce pain when touched.

2. Once you find them, press into the trigger points for 90 seconds until the pain has diminished or gone away. You may have to do several cycles of 90 seconds to accomplish this.

3. Complete normalization of the inner thigh is necessary because this muscle is a major culprit in creating dysfunction and pain in the PFMs and it also contributes to bladder symptoms such as urgency and pain.

External PFMs Trigger Point Therapy for Superficial Transverse Perineal Muscle, Ischiocavernosus Muscle, Bulbospongiosus, Levator Ani, and Perineal Body

External trigger points located anywhere in the low back, hips and legs, and perineal area can refer pain to clitoris, vulva, anus or cause a deep ache in the pelvis. Manipulating and shutting down these external trigger points will bring you a tremendous amount of relief. Many times we are chasing our pain only to discover that it's really coming from another body part. Listed in the charts that follow you will find the most common external trigger points. The charts are divided into body areas, locations of muscle and common referred symptoms. The information in the charts is not only based on hard science but on my clinical experience. I have learned to expect the unexpected.

Keeping this in mind, I have listed what my patients have reported to me regarding their trigger point therapy experience. These external trigger points are so powerful that they can reproduce symptoms such as vulvar pain even though you are not touching that area. Your mission, if you choose to accept it (and I recommend that you do accept it and do not overlook this very important part of your treatment program), is to shut down these trigger points. Eliminate them all by gently pressing into them for 90 seconds or more. The pressure has to be sustained and merciless but within your pain tolerance. Bear in mind that it can take several tries to shut down these trigger points, so don't despair if you don't succeed on your first attempt.

To make long-lasting healing changes in these trigger points can be tricky and can take time. Trigger point therapy can reduce pain by allowing a muscle to come out of its contracted and shortened state to a more normal and lengthened state. When the muscles have their normal length and movement, they get stronger and are less painful. To treat trigger points there needs to be consistent pressure of the moderate-to-heavy kind. But you must work within your pain tolerance and not overdo it. Initially with this kind of pressure your pain will increase, and as the muscle relaxes the pain will subside. The pressure applied to the trigger point should be gradual and when you release the pressure it should also be done slowly. Avoid taking your finger off the trigger point too quickly because the muscle can go into spasm again.

We will first cover the PFMs trigger points. Look at the diagram of the PFMs below and use that as a guide to locate the trigger points. For the body trigger points you will take a look at the muscle location diagram. Acquaint yourself with both these diagrams before starting on your external trigger point therapy work.

PFMS External Trigger Point Therapy

You can have access to the PFMs externally at the perineal area. The area in Diagram 10.3 gives you a great perspective on which PFMs can be accessed externally. Note that the diagram makes the area look larger than it really is. The muscles in this area are close together so keep that in mind when you are looking for the PFMs trigger points. The area in this diagram is also called the perineum. At first you might not be able to neatly discern all the muscles but with practice and by using a mirror while you do the trigger point therapy work you will be able to pinpoint the muscles.

Diagram 10.3: Perineum and External Genitalia

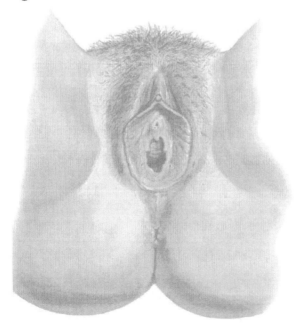

Source: Netter Images

For this therapy pick one of the muscles listed in Table 10.2 and explore it until you find the painful trigger points. Remember that sometimes when you press a trigger point it can refer pain to another area or re-create your symptoms or another symptom. Pay attention and track your pain and symptoms. Draw a map of this area and keep track of your symptoms and pain.

Diagram 10.4: 1st Layer of Pelvic Floor

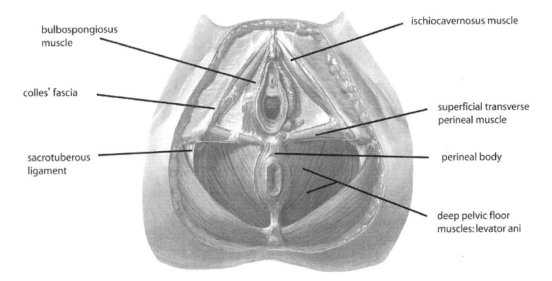

bulbospongiosus muscle

colles' fascia

sacrotuberous ligament

ischiocavernosus muscle

superficial transverse perineal muscle

perineal body

deep pelvic floor muscles: levator ani

Diagram Description: Notice the labeling of the different parts of the first layer of PFMs. Use this diagram as a blueprint to locate your trigger points. Notice that the levator ani muscles take up a lot of the space in the perineum. The levator ani is actually in the 3rd layer of the PFMs but can be seen in this 1st layer diagram. Source of Base Image: Netter Images.

Table 10.2: Pelvic Floor Muscle Trigger Points and Referral Pain Patterns

Refer to Diagram 10.3 and 10.4 for Location of these External PFMs.

PFMS TRIGGER POINTS	REFERRAL PAIN AND/OR SYMPTOMS
Superficial Transverse Perineal Muscle	• Pain at vulva • Pain at site • Pain with sitting • Generalized pelvic pain
Ischiocavernosus Muscle	• Pain at vulva • Perineal pain • Labia pain • Pain with orgasms • Difficulty with orgasms
Bulbospongiosis	• Base at vulva • Perineal pain • Pain with orgasms
Levator Ani (in the ischiorectal fascia)	• Deep pelvic pain • Pain at the site itself • Deep hip pain • Groin pain
Perineal Body	• Rectal pain • Pain at the site itself • Deeper pelvic pain

External Body Trigger Point Therapy

If I had ten dollars for every time I found my patient's pain and symptoms outside the PFMs, I could probably retire. Just because it feels as if the pain is in the pelvis and PFMs does not mean the problem is there. You have to explore your body and become an expert on where your trigger points like to hide. Trigger points are smart and they can be found almost anywhere in the body. For our purposes we will focus on the lower extremity, gluteal and abdominal area and some bone areas. Make sure to work with trigger points as described and instructed throughout this chapter. Refer to both the guideline list and also to the introductory paragraph under external trigger point therapy when working on your trigger points. I encourage you to keep track of the locations where you find your arsenal of trigger points so that you can create a reference map. With a map it is easier to double-check to see if the trigger points are truly gone.

Diagram 10.5: Female Body – Anterior Muscles

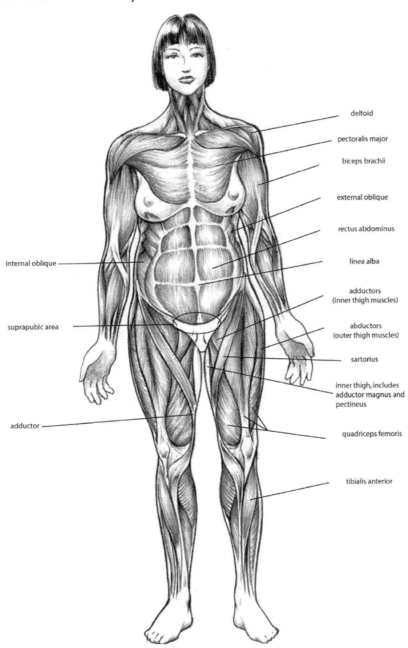

deltoid

pectoralis major

biceps brachii

external oblique

rectus abdominus

internal oblique

linea alba

adductors
(inner thigh muscles)

suprapubic area

abductors
(outer thigh muscles)

sartorius

inner thigh, includes
adductor magnus and
pectineus

adductor

quadriceps femoris

tibialis anterior

Diagram 10.6: Female Body – Posterior Muscles

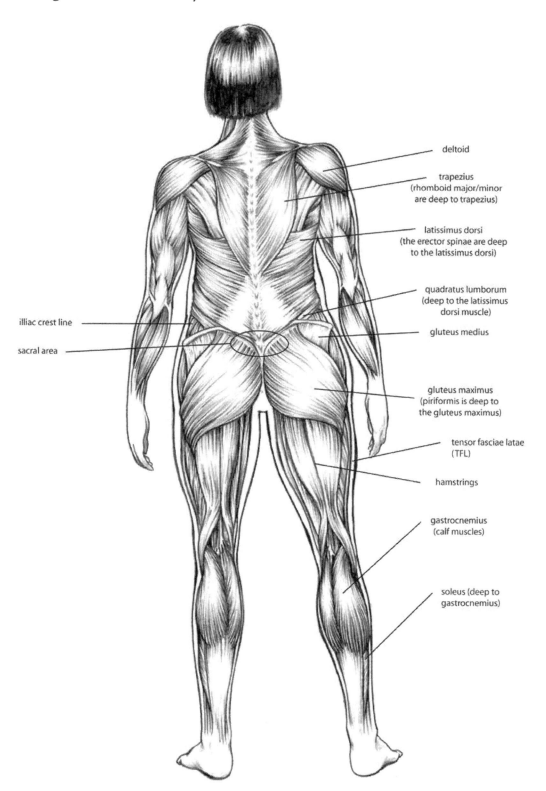

deltoid

trapezius
(rhomboid major/minor
are deep to trapezius)

latissimus dorsi
(the erector spinae are deep
to the latissimus dorsi)

quadratus lumborum
(deep to the latissimus
dorsi muscle)

gluteus medius

iliac crest line

sacral area

gluteus maximus
(piriformis is deep to
the gluteus maximus)

tensor fasciae latae
(TFL)

hamstrings

gastrocnemius
(calf muscles)

soleus (deep to
gastrocnemius)

Table 10.3: Abdominal External Muscular Trigger Point Therapy

MUSCLE TRIGGER POINT LOCATION	BODY LOCATION	SYMPTOMS
Rectus Abdominis	This is the six-pack abdominal muscle. Runs from below the breast bone to the pubic bone. There are two sides, one to the right of the belly button and one to the left.	• Groin/hip pain • Perineum pain • Rectal pain • Suprapubic pain/ bladder pain/ urgency • Labia pain
External Oblique Abdominal	This is the most lateral anterior abdominal muscle, also the largest and most superficial muscle. Usually delineated in women by a line that runs down the outside part of the abdominals.	• Suprapubic pain • Groin pain • Vulvar pain • Perineum pain
Internal Oblique	This muscle is below the external oblique but above the transverse deep abdominal muscle.	• Bladder symptoms • Urgency • General pelvic and rectal symptoms • Pain at site
Suprapubic Abdominal Muscles	This is an area, not really a muscle. This is the abdominal muscle area that resides on top of the pubic bone and is frequently loaded with trigger points that contribute to bladder symptoms.	• Bladder symptoms • Urgency symptoms • Bladder pain
Psoas Muscles (read the psoas section in this chapter to learn how to release trigger points in the psoas)	This is deep muscle that cannot be seen from the outside of the body. It comes from lumbar spine and inserts into the top of leg bone.	• Perineal and vulvar pain • Groin pain • Thigh pain • Knee pain • Low back pain • Bladder symptoms • Bladder pain • Deep ache in the pelvis

Table10.4: Lower Body External Muscular Trigger Point Therapy

MUSCLE TRIGGER POINT LOCATION	BODY LOCATION	SYMPTOMS
Adductor Magnus/Inner Thigh Muscles	Part of the inner thigh muscles; it is biggest and the most medial inner thigh muscle.	• Perineum pain • Vulvar pain • Rectal pain • Groin pain • Bladder symptoms (urgency and frequency of urination)
Pectineus	It is part of the inner thigh muscles and it's the most anterior inner thigh muscle.	• Groin pain • Bladder symptoms
Quadriceps	The big thigh muscle located anterior from the top of the leg to just below the knee.	• Thigh pain • Knee pain • Groin pain • Perineal pain
Hamstrings	The big thigh muscle located posterior from the top of the leg to just below the knee.	• Posterior thigh pain that can travel to the back of the knee • Low back pain • Sacroiliac pain • Sitting pain
Obturator Internus (external access)	Find your sit bone and go medially to the sit bone. To make sure you are on the right muscle resist external rotation of the femur and the muscle pops into your hand.	• Bladder symptoms • Sciatic symptoms • Sitting pain • Deep pelvic pain • Urethral pain • Rectal symptoms • Pudendal neuralgia pain
Coccyx and ligaments	This bone is found above the anus and in between the gluteal muscles.	• Vulvar pain • Deep pelvic pain • Sitting pain • Rectal pain
Piriformis	This muscle is located in the gluteal area. Draw an imaginary line from mid-sacral area to the hip bone and there you will find this muscle.	• Sciatica symptoms • Posterior leg pain • Gluteal pain • Pelvic pain • Sacral pain • Tailbone pain

Table 10.5: Upper Body and Bone Areas External Trigger Point Therapy

MUSCLE TRIGGER POINT LOCATION	BODY LOCATION	SYMPTOMS
Paraspinal back muscle	Located on either side of the spine bones. Pain is usually localized and at the same level as the paraspinal muscle but the lower paraspinal muscles can refer to the gluteal and hip area.	• Pain anywhere on the back area • Gluteal pain • Sit bone pain • Top of hip pain • Sacroiliac pain
Quadratus Lumborum	This muscle can be found posterior in between the lower ribs and the top of the hip bone but lateral to the paraspinal muscles. Once you are in this area you have to press in toward the spine to find the trigger point.	• Groin pain • Labia pain • Hip pain • Sacral pain • Gluteal pain • Sciatica-like pain down the posterior leg
Sacral Area	This is not a muscle but an area that frequently can have trigger points. This area can be found in the middle of the two butt cheeks. It is a diamond- shaped area and houses some of the nerves that give life to the PFMs and it also has gluteal muscles that attach to it. You can either perform trigger point therapy at the edges of the sacrum or do sacral rolling. This area houses sacral nerve S2 to S4.	• Sacroiliac joint pain • Gluteal pain • Bladder symptoms • Urgency symptoms • Perineal pain • Vulvar pain
Iliac Crest Line	This is not a muscle but an area where many muscles live. So investigating this top hip crease line will bring relief.	• Localized low back pain • Gluteal pain • Hip pain • Sacroiliac joint pain
Greater Trochanter of the Femur (posterior and anterior aspects)	This is not a muscle but a very important area that tends to have trigger points. Many of the posterior hip muscles insert into this bone. Imagine that the back of the bone is a clock. Press at each point of the clock not only in the front but the back aspect of the bone itself to release pain. Can use a tennis ball here to help release these trigger points.	• Vulvar pain • Leg pain • Pelvic pain • Hip pain • Back pain
Sit Bones	The bones that we sit on. These bones have surrounding fascia that are intimately connected with the gluteal and hip muscles. Imagine these bones like clocks. Go around each bone and find trigger points that are painful.	• Pain with sitting • Deep pelvic ache/pain

Table 10.6: Gluteal Muscles External Body Trigger Point Therapy

MUSCLE TRIGGER POINT LOCATION	BODY LOCATION	SYMPTOMS
Gluteus Maximus	The biggest and most superficial of the gluteal butt muscles.	• Tailbone pain • Buttock pain • Rectal pain • Hip pain • Sit bone pain and pain with sitting • Sacral pain • Posterior thigh pain
Gluteus Medius	This is a gluteal muscle that is under the gluteus maximus and can be found to the outside of the butt cheek near the top of the hip bone.	• Perineum pain • Labia pain • Hip pain • Sciatica-like symptoms • Posterior thigh pain
Gluteus Minimus	This is the smallest and innermost of the gluteal muscles. It lies under the gluteus medius muscle.	• Labia pain • Pain down the posterior thigh • Pain with sitting • Buttock pain
Tensor Fascia Latae (TFL)	Comes from the side of the hip bone, runs on the outside of the thigh and inserts into the knee. Look for trigger points not only on the TFL but to the outer sides of it.	• Hip pain • Lateral thigh pain • Knee pain • Pain with walking and running • Difficulty lying on the affected side • Pain going from sitting to standing

Strain-Counterstrain(S/CS) for Obturator Internus

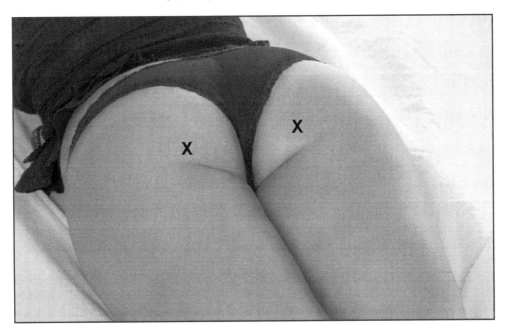

Description: Please note the above photo only shows the location of the sit bones. The exercise below is performed on your stomach.

Strain-counterstrain techniques can have dramatic pain-relieving effects for those suffering from pelvic, hip, and gluteal pain. I have found that when I use these techniques as part of my patients' treatment sessions they often get immediate relief, and have better mobility and improved range of motion in stubborn, tight muscles.

The strain-counterstrain technique was developed by Dr. Lawrence Jones, an osteopathic doctor. It is a gentle and safe technique that passively shortens the affected muscle areas by holding those muscles in a contracted state for 90 seconds. When the muscle is held in this position, it gradually returns to its original resting position and length and is therefore less painful. It's pretty easy to do as part of your self-care as well. These techniques are great to use with a partner, but you can also just use them on your own with some modifications. I have included the top two that I think are the easiest to do on yourself and that could give you the most pain relief.

Always grade your pain on a scale of 0 to 10. Grading your pain this way tracks your progress to see if your pain is improving. Remember that it is important to come out of this position slowly and mindfully.

Obturator Internus S/CS Techniques

Obturator internus (OI) pain is very common in women with pelvic pain and PFM dysfunction. Trigger points and/or spasms located in this muscle can also refer pain to the pelvic and hip area. A great technique that quiets this muscle down is the strain-counterstrain technique. Although the OI muscle is an external rotator of the hip, it can be accessed either intravaginally or externally. You can hurt yourself with this technique if you press too hard into this area.

WHAT TO DO:

1. Lie on your stomach, find your right sit bone with your right hand and go slightly medial to it, toward the inside of the bone. Press inward toward the right sit bone and look for painful spots. This is where the trigger point is commonly found for the OI. Be very gentle in this area. Do not press hard.

2. While holding the spot with your right hand, bend your right knee to 90 degrees and allow the foot to fall inward, producing external rotation of the hip. The OI muscle will "pop" into your hand.

3. Hold the spot with the knee bent and lower leg rotated inward for 90 seconds and retest to see if your pain has decreased. Repeat on the left side.

4. This is a long sustained hold while the OI is in max contraction.

Contract/Relax for Obturator Internus

Description: Please note the above photo only shows the location of the sit bones. The exercise below is performed on your stomach.

WHAT TO DO:

1. Lie on your stomach, find your right sit bone with your right hand and go slightly medial to it, toward the inside of the bone. Press inward toward the right sit bone and look for painful spots. This is where the trigger point is commonly found for the OI.

2. While holding the spot with your right hand, bend your right knee to 90 degrees. Keep the knee bent at neutral or you can keep the leg straight. Contract your gluteal/butt muscles for 10 to 15 seconds and then relax for 10 to 15 seconds. Repeat five to ten times.

3. The pain at the spot that you are touching should be decreasing. If the pain is increasing, stop this technique or re-examine what you are doing. The goal is to have less pain in the trigger point area, not more.

Psoas Release

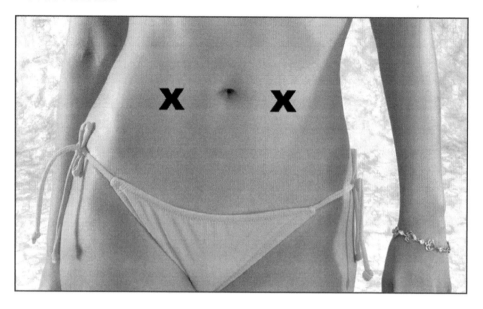

Your body has two very deep muscles on either side of the lower abdomen called the psoas muscles. These muscles attach from the lower spine to the hip bones, and help flex the hips. The psoas muscles are frequently very painful, in spasm, and irritated in women suffering from pelvic pain. This technique is highly effective in reducing pain and normalizing PFMs tension and function. Psoas release is also great for women who have low back pain.

To find the psoas muscles do the following:

1. Lie on your back with your legs straight out.

2. Go about two to three inches to the right side of your belly button. Place your fingertips into the area, slowly allowing them to sink into your abdomen and being careful to avoid any feelings of an artery pulse.

3. Lift your right leg straight up and you will feel the psoas pop into your hand. It may take a little practice to get this but keep trying. Once you know where the psoas muscle is, place your fingertips in that spot and slowly press

downward into the psoas for 60 to 90 seconds. If you feel any tingling, numbness, or tremendous increase in pain, get off the area and try to relocate the psoas muscle. Switch sides and do the left psoas muscle release.

4. CAUTION HERE: Do not press into an area that has a pulse. If you feel a pulse, move to a different area and locate the muscle at another place.

Proprioceptive Neuromuscular Techniques (PNF) Contract/Relax for Global PFMs Relaxation

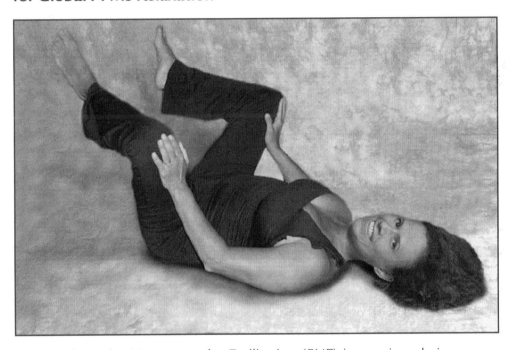

Proprioceptive Neuromuscular Facilitation (PNF) isometric techniques can help release tension in the pelvic floor muscles naturally. The following PNF pattern works particularly well to help maintain a relaxed state in the PFMs.

WHAT TO DO:

1. Lie on your back with your knees bent and aligned with your hips so that your hips and knees form a right angle.

2. Place your hands on the top of your knees, allowing your knees to move outward, as in the photo.

3. As you exhale, press your hands into your knees and your knees into your hands, giving yourself resistance, but not allowing the position to change.

4. The line of force is going to be toward your shoulders, but don't let your hands or legs move.

5. Release the tension on your thighs and then concentrate on feeling the relaxation of the PFMs and then try to perform a reverse Kegel. Perform the reverse Kegel up to ten seconds.

6. Hold the resistance for ten seconds, rest for ten seconds, repeat three times per set, two to three times per day. Focus on the reverse Kegel exercise.

Diagram 10.7: Location of the Anal Rim

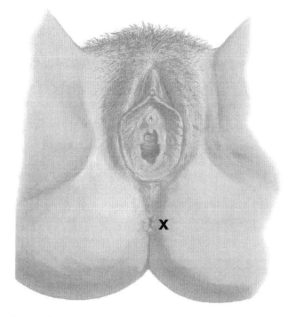

Source: Netter Images

Anal Rim Massage

Many of my female patients cannot wrap their heads around the intrarectal work. I understand their resistance. The intrarectal pelvic floor muscle therapy is not comfortable and can be painful. I usually start patients off with touching and massaging the skin outside of the anus. The massage is done around the rim of the entire anus with gentle pressure. You would be amazed how many of my patients get pain relief from this simple technique. It can help women suffering from anal pain and/or constipation.

WHAT TO DO:

1. Spread the buttocks to reveal the anus.

2. Slowly and gently massage the rim using circular motions in a clockwise direction only.

3. You can use some type of organic oil for this massage.

4. You can massage the anal rim for three to five minutes or as tolerated. Get as close to the anus as possible. If you have external hemorrhoids this technique might not be for you. Proceed with caution or don't do it at all. Rubbing external hemorrhoids might cause them to bleed or get worse.

Suprapubic External Bladder Trigger Points

Many of my patients complain about pain right above the pubic bone. The bladder and some of the PFMs live underneath this pubic bone. If there is a dysfunction, these muscles and organs could refer pain to the top of the pubic bone and the lower abdominal area. This next technique brings about amazing results and can help reduce bladder urgency. Many times trigger points in this area cause bladder pain and pain with urination. This is one of my go-to techniques for women suffering from bladder conditions.

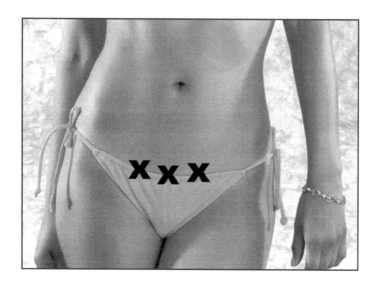

WHAT TO DO:

1. Start your investigation by pressing along the top of the pubic bone and your lower abdominal muscle area. Take note of where the pain is and what symptoms you feel when you press into these areas.

2. Make yourself a simple map. Note pain level from 0 to 10 (0 = no pain, 10 = worst pain) and symptoms produced.

3. Hold the trigger point for 90 seconds, making sure to release the trigger point slowly. Repeat as many times as necessary until the pain level is reduced by 50 percent or you feel relief from the symptoms.

4. CAUTION HERE: Do not press into an area that has a pulse. If you feel a pulse, move to a different area.

Diagram 10.8: Location of the Perineum

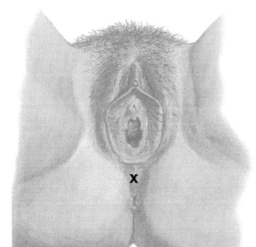

Diagram Description: Notice that the perineal area is very small. Imagine the clock positions in this small area. The X marks the perineal body and perineum. Source: Netter Images

Perineum Pressure Point Technique

The perineum is the area between the vagina and the anus. In some pelvic surgeries and during childbirth this area can get traumatized. The site where episiotomies are frequently performed, this is a big source of pain for new moms who have experienced a perineal tear. Many times you can relieve pelvic pain by working and finding trigger points in this area. If you've had a surgery you will need to get medical clearance before doing this technique. It will be important for you to address this area because of the scar tissue that many times results after surgeries and childbirth.

WHAT TO DO:

1. Start your investigation by pressing along the perineal area. Take note of where the pain is and what symptoms you feel when you press into these areas.

2. Make yourself a simple map. Note pain level from 0 to 10 (0 = no pain, 10 = worst pain) and symptoms produced. Think of the perineum as a clock as you did with other techniques.

3. For best results, try pressing into the perineal body at different angles and locations in the perineum. Hold each different direction for up to 90 seconds or as tolerated. The goal is to promote flexibility and to decrease pain and/or symptoms by 50 percent.

Basic Clitoral Anatomy

A source of fascination for many, the clitoris has been poorly described and understood. When I started researching this area, I noticed that the anatomic descriptions of the clitoris varied. Many of my patients who suffer from pelvic pain complain about clitoral pain, clitoral hypersensitivity and/or clitoral hyposensitivity. In this section we will review the anatomy of the clitoris; it plays a profound part in female pelvic pain conditions and responds well to manual clitoral hood release or stretch.

The clitoris, a female sex organ, is a multi-planar and three-dimensional structure and reaches deep within the female pelvis. It is neither flat, nor pointed nor straight but expansive and deeply connected to the vaginal wall, pubic bone, urethra and PFMs. The clitoris is located deep to smaller vaginal lips called the labia minora and slightly above the opening of the urethra (where urine exits the body). Unlike the penis, the clitoris maintains a bent position via its supportive ligaments. When the clitoris becomes aroused it can become engorged and swollen much like a penis does. The clitoris can also increase in size, become erect and increase in sensitivity with sexual desire. The clitoris is not just one simple organ but a complex that lives inside and outside the female body. Most of the clitoris is located inside the body and cannot be seen. The anatomy of this structure has been under scrutiny and has become better understood with the help of urologist

Helen O'Connell. Thanks to her research and MRI studies we have discovered wonderful things about the clitoris. The clitoris contains many different parts and is intimately connected to other female structures within the pelvis.

The clitoris is large and has several parts that include the glans of clitoris, body or shaft of clitoris, paired crura, paired bulbs or vestibules, and the paired corpus cavernosa (together form the corpus cavernosum). The glans of clitoris is an extension of the body of the clitoris (internal clitoris) and is partly on the outside. The glans is said to contain 8,000 sensory nerves. Many believe that the glans is the clitoris because it sticks out but it's only a subpart of the whole thing. We see the glans of clitoris on the outside, so for a long time many scientists and doctors thought this was the clitoris.

The body or shaft of the clitoris is inside the body. The clitoral shaft/body is a deeper more embedded structure that attaches to the undersurface of the pubic bone. The body of the clitoris is made up of two corpus cavernosa. It's a spongy tissue that houses a lot of blood and thereby enhances clitoral erections. When

Diagram 10.9: Basic Anatomy of the Clitoris

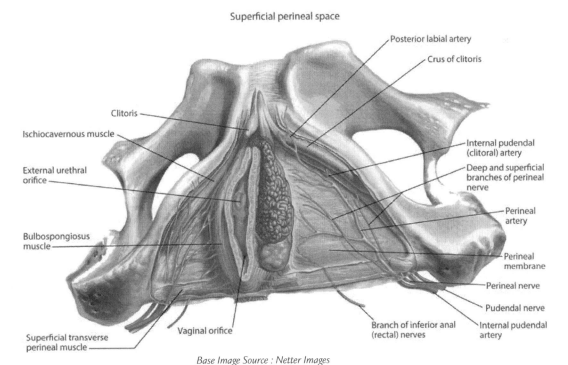

Base Image Source : Netter Images

erect, the corpus carvernosa surrounds the vagina on either side as if giving the vagina a big hug.

The corpus cavernosum divides further and become the crura of the clitoris which also contains a high level of erectile tissue. The crura are laterally located and are associated with the ischiocavernosus, one of the superficial pelvic floor muscles. It is important to note here that the superficial PFMs, the bulbospongiosus and ischiocarvernosus muscle, insert into the clitoris and overlie erectile tissue playing an important role in female sexual function and clitoral erection. The paired crura have a wishbone shape and some call them the legs of the clitoris. The crura come together at the body and attach themselves to the pubic bone. The clitoral bulbs (vestibule) are located on either side of the clitoral body medially to the clitoral crura. The clitoral bulbs (vestibule) are underneath the labia minora next to the vaginal opening.

Diagram 10.10: Location of the CLitoral Hood

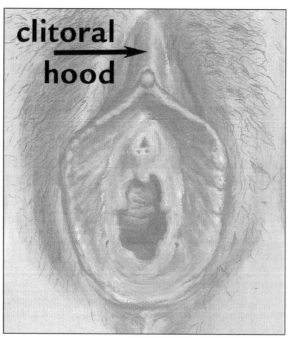

The clitoral hood protects the clitoral gland and should move freely. Sometimes women experience adhesions of the clitoral hood and the hood can get bound down. This lack of movement in the clitoral hood can be a major cause of clitoral pain. In this next section I will provide you

Source: Netter Images

with a technique to free up the clitoral hood. Many women who suffer from clitoral pain complain of clitoral itching, excessive swelling and pain. Clitoral pain can be experienced with or without direct clitoral contact. Many believe that malfunctioning of its nerves can be one of the main causes of clitoral pain. Some women experience the opposite; instead of clitoral pain, there's an overarousal and spontaneous uncontrolled sexual arousal present. This response is not like normal sexual arousal. This hypersexual response can be troublesome for many women because it is not associated with sexual desire and can persist for hours, days or off and on. This condition is called Persistent Sexual Arousal Syndrome (PSAD) and is not associated with a hypersexual drive or being promiscuous. Sometimes PSAD is associated with pudendal nerve neuralgia or pudendal nerve entrapment.

Clitoral Hood Release and Stretch Overview

GETTING STARTED:

As previously stated, these clitoral techniques are great for women suffering from clitoral pain and hypo- or hypersensitivity of the clitoris with or without sexual dysfunction. They must be performed very gently and without causing pain. Many times the clitoral hood is bound down and not moving freely as it should. In these cases the releases and stretches have be performed extra carefully to avoid micro-trauma to the tissue. The hood should move freely. If it doesn't, don't despair. Just work on the hood until it becomes mobile and free.

Clitoral Hood Release

WHAT TO DO:

Locate your clitoris by following your labia minora upward until you have located the glans of the clitoris (external part). The hood covers the glans clitoris. Imagine the top part of the hood as a clock. Twelve o'clock is at the middle, 1 o'clock to the left and 11 o'clock to the right. Gently place your index finger at the 12 o'clock position and gently move the hood slightly upward. Hold for 3 to 5 seconds or as tolerated. Now repeat the same process at the 11 o'clock and 1 o'clock positions. Repeat two to three times at each clock point. Monitor for pain and avoid pain levels over three. Use a mirror to see where the clitoral hood is moving or not moving and so that you can track your progress.

Clitoral Hood Stretch

WHAT TO DO:

Once the hood is freed up and moving well you can start to incorporate the clitoral hood stretching. Locate your clitoris by following your labia minora upward until you have located the glans of the clitoris (external part). Place your one index finger at the 12 o'clock position above the glans but on the superior part of the clitoral hood. Place the other index finger on the upper part of the labia minora but below the glans clitoris. Maintaining a firm sustained pressure on the labia minora pull the hood gently upward towards the pubic bone until you feel a gentle stretch. Hold for up to 10 seconds or as tolerated. Repeat 2 to 3 times.

This chapter is definitely intense, but this intensity can bring great rewards. Please go slowly as you work with the powerful techniques discussed here. Track your responses so that you can piece together which tools are having the best effect on your symptoms.

In the next chapter we go in and fine tune our techniques for scar therapy and manipulation. There are many tools to choose from in this upcoming chapter, so remember to take your time and first get clearance from your MD before starting a scar and adhesion therapy program.

Chapter Eleven

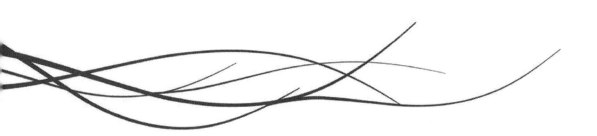

"Worry pretends to be necessary
but serves no useful purpose."
- Eckhart Tolle

Chapter 11

SCAR-CARE TECHNIQUES

As outlined in Chapter 2, post-surgical scar adhesions occur in women after most pelvic, abdominal, and C-section surgeries. The fibrous bands that form during the healing process post surgery often cause tissues to grow together that normally would not be connected. In my experience, the longer a woman waits to seek therapy for her scars, the denser and tougher the scar adhesions become. I have seen women develop pelvic and sexual pain as a result of abdominal surgeries for fibroids, hysterectomy, C-sections, and endometriosis, even though there were no incisions made in the pelvic floor muscles.

New mothers are one group of women that tend to be overlooked and often not even classified as post-operative. I treat many post-partum women at my healing center who have had significant perineal tears or episiotomies during their labor, who then come to me complaining about sexual pain. Their common complaint is that they are not "the same down there." Sometimes they tell me their husbands no longer fit inside them. Many of these new mothers have significant sexual pain, pain with walking, and/or pain with sitting. Recent research has shown that one out of three women have sexual pain a year after giving birth. Many of these young mothers also complain that they have trouble with breastfeeding and taking care of their young infants because of their abdominal or perineal scar pain. Many patients tell me that they have heard there is nothing you can do to alleviate these conditions, and are often told things like "Welcome to motherhood."

Another group of women often overlooked are those who have undergone C-sections. The statistics show that over 31 percent of births in the US are done by C-section. Make no mistake: a C-section is a major surgery. Adhesions, pelvic and sexual pain are often a direct result of scars that have become bound down. I often see C-section patients who have developed vulvodynia and pelvic floor muscle dysfunction as a result of the surgery.

Women who have experienced any of the above surgical procedures will benefit from stretching and mobilizing their scars to prevent scar adhesions. Many women who come to me have no idea how to care for their scars. In particular women who undergo C-sections or other abdominal surgeries are often not given advice on how to care for their scars when they leave the hospital. Some may even feel ashamed of their C-section scars because they feel a sense of failure over not having the vaginal birth.

Many women are afraid to touch their scars and experience problems because their scars are bound down, inflexible and have multiple dense adhesions. Furthermore, post-surgical patients often complain to me about upper and lower back and neck pain. I find many of these spinal pains are related to postural problems because their scars are pulling their bodies inward and forward, causing trigger points and spasms in the scars and muscles. Some of my patients also complain about not being able to wear certain clothes. Many tell me they feel changes in the weather in their scars. The critical thing to remember is that post-surgical scars must be dealt with and that scar pain and adhesions must be resolved as part of the solution in the journey to regain normal functioning and pain-free intimacy.

Before undertaking any of the scar therapy techniques in this chapter, it is critical to look at Table 11.1 for warning signs and precautions. Make sure to check with your doctor or birth caregiver to get their approval before starting any of the scar techniques and massages. When in doubt about a technique, seek help from a healthcare professional such as a physical therapist who specializes in pelvic floor and scar conditions to make sure you get on the right track.

In Their Own Words - Post-Partum Scar Pain; 4th-Degree Tear

"I came to Renew Physical Therapy to see Isa because I had post-partum scar pain from 3 surgical repairs. During the birth of my child I experienced a 4th-degree tear to my perineum and rectum. I felt very weak and wanted to be stronger. My doctor said I was perfectly healed, but I was still in so much pain. He said this was normal and to be expected, so I believed him. For 2 months I tried to ignore the pain, so when I came to see Isa and she asked me if I had any pain, I said no. I really wasn't connected to my pelvic muscles, so I thought I had no pain.

"Isa taught me how to keep track of my pain in a journal even though I told her I just came to retrain and strengthen my muscles. With my journal on hand at my next appointment, I realized that not only did I have pain, but I had extreme pain all day, in every situation! I had pain with sitting and had pain with sex. Wearing my thong underwear also hurt.

"I have been seeing Isa for about 2 months now and she worked with me to strengthen, stretch and mobilize my scar tissue. We worked both on the vaginal and rectal tissues. She used laser therapy as well which was amazing, I literally walked out of the healing center with no pain the first time she did it. Each time after that, I just got better and better. Now, after 2 months, I feel stronger than even before I had my son. I am almost pain-free. I am able to wear clothes without any difficulty, including my tight jeans and thong underwear without pain.

"I highly recommend physical therapy at Renew PT for women who have had a baby – whether they were injured or not or had a C-section or not - to get better and stronger. A lot of times, we are unaware of what is happening in our bodies until someone focuses on it. I am really thankful for Renew Physical Therapy."

Table 11.1: Precautions for Abdominal and Perineal Scar Therapy

TYPE OF PRECAUTION
1. If you have recently had surgery, get clearance from your medical doctor before starting the vaginal and abdominal techniques in this chapter.
2. If you have recently given birth and have an episiotomy, perineal tear and/or perineal repair, get clearance from your midwife or medical doctor before starting the vaginal techniques, dilator stretches or abdominal scar therapy outlined in this chapter.
3. Proceed with caution if you have undergone abdominal surgeries. Check with your doctor to make sure that the scar therapy and massage techniques in this book are appropriate for your recovery.
4. Avoid the techniques in this chapter if you have a vaginal infection, abdominal scar infection or bleeding from the vagina or abdominal scar.
5. Avoid abdominal scar massage if your scar is oozing fluids. Inform your caregiver about any changes to your scars.
6. If you have recently given birth, wait 6 weeks before massaging perineal and Cesarian section scars and get medical clearance first from your midwife or doctor.
7. Report any increase in scar pain to your caregiver, and have your doctor check to make sure the scar is healing well.
8. Immediately report to your caregiver any foul-smelling odor coming from your vagina, abdominal or perineal scar as this could be a sign of infection.
9. Always start gently and superficially with all massage techniques listed in this chapter. Discontinue if the scar becomes painful.
10. I recommend getting expert advice from a women's health physiotherapist to make sure you are performing the techniques correctly.
11. You can massage the scar as soon as the Steri-Strips fall off. Only massage the areas of the scar that are healed completely. Don't massage parts of the scar that are open or oozing.
12. If you are unsure about the techniques, wait until your 6 week checkup before starting or continuing the techniques in this chapter.

Scar Massage Therapy Basics

Massaging scars, whether in the perineum or abdominal area, helps to restore proper function to the muscles, increase blood circulation to the muscles, promote better scar healing, and prevent adhesions from becoming too tough or dense. If you have a C-section scar, a myomectomy or other abdominal scar, it is usually alright to start gently massaging an abdominal scar as soon as the Steri-Strips have fallen off, and you have approval from your doctor.

If you have any doubts about massaging the scar, consult your physician and/or caregiver about when to start. Different surgical procedures heal at different rates. Many doctors have their own protocols as to when the scar therapy can start. You will always derive benefits with proper massage of your scar, but YOU MUST GET CLEARANCE from your doctor BEFORE STARTING any scar massage techniques to avoid altering the surgical procedure and possibly damaging the tissues. For these scar massage techniques, you can use massage cream once your doctor or caregiver gives the green light. You can also use scar oils or ointments such as Mederma, scar guard, vitamin E, or even plain olive oil to do your massages.

Table 11.2: Scar Therapy Techniques for the Relief of Pain and Adhesions

TECHNIQUE
1. Scar Trigger Point Release
2. Abdominal Scar Massage Long Strokes
3. Deeper Scar Massage: Clockwise Circles
4. Abdominal Scar Lift
5. Abdominal Scar Rolling
6. Scar Stretching Techniques – Longitudinal
7. Scar Down and X-Pattern
8. Perineal/Vaginal Massage Therapy

Scar Trigger Point Release

WHAT TO DO:

1. Check the length of the scar and press gently along it looking for spots that elicit pain when touched or that refer pain to another location.

2. Once a painful spot is found, gently press into it, holding the spot without releasing the pressure for 60 to 90 seconds. Repeat 2 to 3 times until the pain has diminished. Repeat the point pressure therapy several times until the scar pain is reduced by 50 percent. You can apply pressure on the same spot for several 60 to 90 second repetitions until the pain has subsided.

3. Avoid pressing into the scar too aggressively. Grade your pressure and press into the scar to a tolerable pain level. Pressing into the scar too hard will cause the PFM to tighten in response to the scar pain.

4. While you are doing your scar point pressure therapy, pay attention to your pelvic floor muscles and make sure to keep them relaxed. Also, to deal with the pain, it helps to breathe diaphragmatically, with long deep breaths, in through the nose and out through the mouth.

Abdominal Scar Massage Long Strokes

WHAT TO DO:

1. To restore flexibility to an abdominal or C-section scar, massage it using long strokes along the length of the scar.

2. Perform 20 long strokes from left to right across the scar superficially at first and then as the pain decreases, go deeper until you are at the layer of the adhesions.

3. Repeat with 20 long strokes from right to left.

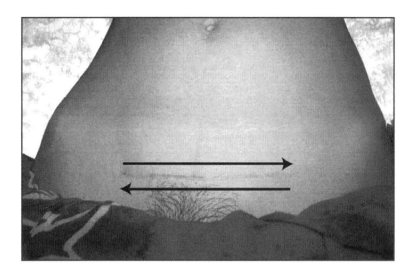

Deeper Scar Massage: Clockwise Circles

WHAT TO DO:

1. Perform small clockwise circles along the scar from right to left, using different graded pressure as tolerated. Start superficially and then go deeper as you are able. Repeat with small circles from left to right.

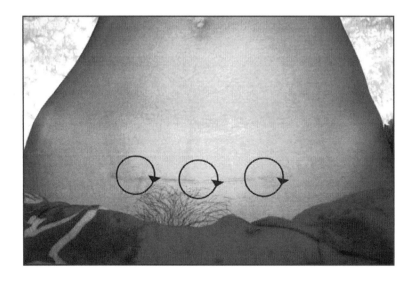

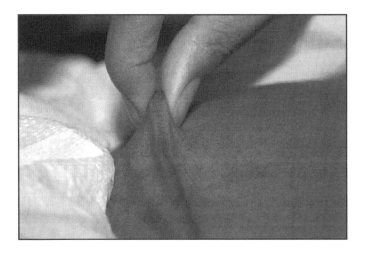

Abdominal Scar Lift

WHAT TO DO:

1. Divide the scar into small areas. Starting on one side, pick up the scar between your index finger and thumb. Try to pick up some of the underlying scar tissue, not just the outer layer of skin.

2. Once you pick up the scar and some of the underlying tissue, hold it for 30 seconds before moving across to the next section. If needed, you can hold the upward lift longer and wait for the scar to release. The release will feel like the scar is lengthening naturally.

Abdominal Scar Rolling

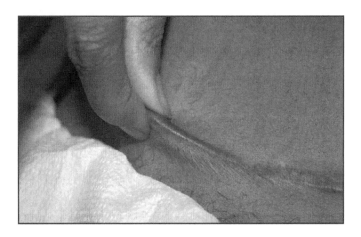

WHAT TO DO:

1. Pick up the scar along its length and roll it between your thumb and index finger. This might be very difficult to do if the scar is bound down or inflexible.

2. If the scar does not lift up, do not be alarmed. Your goal is to break up the adhesions and to be able to lift up the skin of the scar.

Scar Stretching Techniques – Longitudinal, Scar Down, X-Pattern

GETTING STARTED:

Just like other muscles in the body, scars can benefit immensely from being stretched. There are three main types of stretching I recommend to my patients that provide the most relief, but do not attempt to do scar stretching unless you get clearance from your doctor or caregiver.

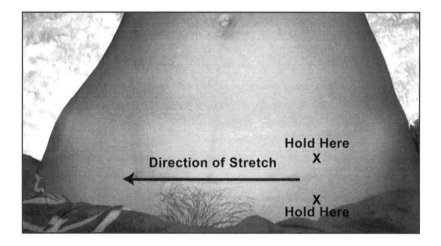

Longitudinal Scar Stretch

WHAT TO DO:

1. Hold down the left side of the scar and with your left hand, stretch the scar by pulling it to the right with your right hand until you feel resistance.

2. Hold the stretch for 30 to 60 seconds.

3. Repeat 2 to 5 times, then switch sides.

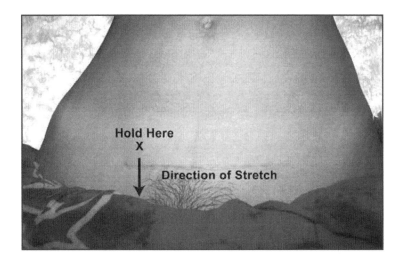

Scar Down Stretch

WHAT TO DO:

1. Place your right index finger on top of the scar about a half inch away from the scar and place your left index finger below the scar in a straight line.

2. Hold the right index finger in place and gently use the left finger to stretch the scar in a linear pattern as if you were trying to pull the scar apart.

3. Continue this stretching along the scar from right to left and from left to right, as shown in the photo.

X Pattern Scar Stretch

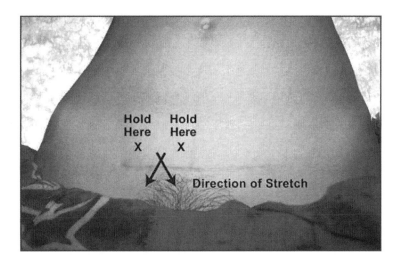

WHAT TO DO:

1. Place your right index finger on top of the scar about a half inch away from the scar and place your left index finger diagonally below the scar.

2. Pull the fingers away from each other, thereby stretching the scar. Hold this stretch for 5 seconds, then switch hands. Place your left index finger above the scar and your right index finger below the scar and pull the fingers away from each other, holding for another 5 seconds.

3. This type of stretching creates an X pattern. Perform this X pattern along the scar first, from right to left and then left to right.

Perineal/Vaginal Massage Therapy

Many of the women I treat have pelvic pain resulting from an episiotomy or a perineal tear during the delivery of their child. When they come to see me they are in a state of depression and anxiety. Not only do they have a newborn at home that requires their undivided attention but now they also have to endure pain while sitting, standing, and in many cases simply changing positions. Other women who can benefit from this type of stretching include those who have undergone biopsies, vestibulodectomy, or reconstructive surgeries.

For the perineal/vaginal scar therapy, it is helpful to use a mirror to look and examine the scar before stretching and mobilizing the scar. The following massage routines are great techniques that can be used to alleviate painful scars in the perineum. These methods can also be used to help mobilize and make the pelvic floor muscles more supple, flexible and pain-free. These techniques work great for women who are on a healing journey to pain-free intimacy, and can be used even if you don't have a scar.

Perineal Scar Rolling (no illustration)

WHAT TO DO:

1. Place the scar between the fingertips. You might have to place one finger inside the vagina and one finger outside the vagina, gently gripping the scar between the fingertips in order to roll it.

2. Roll the scar between your fingers for 2 to 3 minutes or as tolerated until the scar feels loose, less painful and more pliable. Perineal scar rolling is a great method to get the scar more flexible and mobile.

Perineal Body Massage

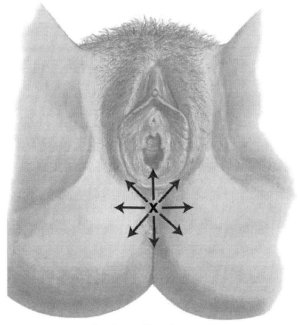

Base Image: Netter Images

WHAT TO DO:

1. Use the trigger point release techniques as outlined earlier in Part III, but this time on the perineal body.

2. Once you locate a painful area or trigger point, push on that spot for 90 seconds.

3. For best results, try pressing into the perineal body at different angles and locations in the perineum. Hold each different direction for 20 to 30 seconds.

Traditional Perineal Thumb Massage

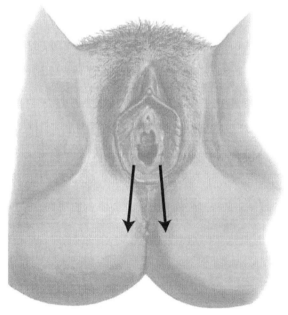

Direction of Thumbs

Base Image: Netter Images

GETTING STARTED:

This massage method works great for perineal scars, for pelvic pain sufferers with vaginismus, and also as a preparation for labor and delivery. Pregnant women can start this massage on the 34th week of pregnancy for 3 to 5 minutes. Make sure to check with your obstetrician, gynecologist or midwife before starting the perineal massage. I often teach my pregnant patients' partners to do this massage to help them prepare for labor.

WHAT TO DO:

1. Lubricate your thumbs, insert them into the vagina up to the first knuckle, and press straight downward towards the rectum for 3 to 5 minutes.

2. After 3 to 5 minutes, press down to the right for several seconds and then to the left for several seconds.

3. Another technique is to do half-moon strokes with your thumbs. Place your right thumb up to the first knuckle in the inside of your left pelvic floor muscles. Start from top to bottom performing half-moon strokes from the top to bottom for about one minute, then change sides and perform the half-moon strokes on the other side.

So far we have covered a lot of ground and I've presented many techniques that you can incorporate as you work hard to reduce your symptoms. Remember, as I mentioned in Part I, you have to get on a road that will transform every aspect of your life. This includes having at your disposal a set of tools and information that you will use in times when you are not stretching, exercising, massaging, and mobilizing your pelvic floor muscles.

The tools and techniques that you will read about next in Part IV are great tips and strategies that can bring soothing comfort and relief for irritated skin, painful flare-ups and muscle spasms. You also need to pull together an all-encompassing mind-body approach with daily meditations, visualizations, and affirmations to break the cycle of self-blame, shame, and hopelessness that often accompanies conditions involving the PFMs.

Again, as in Part III, there is no set order or series outlined in this next section as in the stretching and strengthening series. I have merely put together a pelvic pain relief toolbox for you filled with my most tried and true techniques and remedies that my patients tell me give them the most relief and motivation to continue on their journeys to pain-free living.

Part 4
Pelvic Pain Relief Toolbox

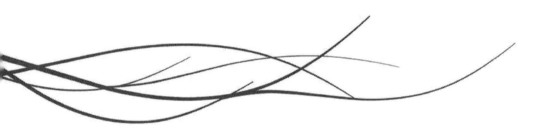

*"Learn from yesterday, live for today,
hope for tomorrow."*
—Albert Einstein

Chapter 12

❦

BASIC TOOLS FOR BETTER VULVAR SKIN CARE

When my patients come to see me at my center I always ask them, "When was the last time you examined your vagina?" Almost always, the answer varies from never to several months. I think it's safe to say that most women are not taught vulva-vaginal health, self-care and self-examination. As a child, the only vulvar care/hygiene I learned was to wipe from front to back. Proper vulvar care, hygiene, and self-examination are great ways to understand your unique anatomy, understand what is normal for you, and are essential in monitoring your vulvar health. The importance of performing monthly vulvar self-exam cannot be stressed enough, which is why I dedicated a whole section of this book in Part I to vaginal self-examination. I've seen several different physicians in the past several years and not once was I instructed on how to do this exam.

Remember, as we discussed in Part I, you will do your self-exam at least once a month and take note of any changes. Track issues like skin irritation, changes in coloration, discharge, pain levels and locations, and any other relevant information that will help you get a better understanding of your pelvic floor. If you are experiencing burning, itching, or irritation, use some of the great remedies listed in this chapter to get some relief. If your condition persists, make sure you work with a doctor who can help make some specific recommendations as well. The techniques I am presenting in this chapter are by no means a substitute for proper medical care.

Basic Vulvar Skin Hygiene

Irritation and burning of the vulva and vagina are common among women suffering from pelvic pain conditions. There are many things you can do to minimize these feelings in your vulva. The following is a list of recommendations that have worked for my patients. Remember, these are only recommendations and you must find the ones that are appropriate for you and your condition. If you have any doubt, please show the list to your caregiver to make sure that you are practicing the ones that will work best for you.

Recommendations for Better Vulvar Care

1. Although it may seem obvious, always wipe from front to back after urination and bowel movement to avoid infections.

2. Keep the vulva area dry. Pat dry the vulva; do not vigorously rub it with towels or toilet paper. If the vulva is irritated, use a blow drier set on cool or let it air dry.

3. Sleep in the nude at night. My patients find sleeping in the nude helps reduce their irritation.

4. Avoid irritants such as perfumed soaps, bubble bath, feminine hygiene products and colored toilet paper on the vulva. If you must use soap, try something gentle and fragrance-free or try calendula soap. Also avoid getting shampoo on the vulva.

5. Use unscented white and chlorine-free toilet paper, and whenever possible, use organic toilet paper.

6. Use menstrual pads and tampons that are perfume-free and 100 percent cotton. Make sure to use the appropriate tampon size for menstrual flow.

During light days, use tampons with lighter absorbency, and during heavy days use super absorbency. Again whenever possible, use organic products and avoid deodorized sanitary pads and tampons.

7. Avoid pushing with urination and defecation. Avoid constipation by drinking enough water for proper hydration and taking in enough fiber. Staying properly hydrated helps keep the urine diluted and makes it less likely to irritate the vulva and the bladder.

8. After urinating, rinse the vulva with cool to lukewarm water. A perineal bottle (spray bottle) works great. Alternatively, you can invest in a bidet for your home. Using a perineal bottle is especially great after childbirth.

9. Avoid douches unless prescribed by your caregiver. Douches can upset the natural balance of organisms in the vagina.

10. Avoid chlorinated water and avoid swimming in pools. I've had patients flare-up terribly after being in chlorinated pools.

11. Perform vaginal steams as described later in Part IV once a week and the day after your menstrual cycle ends.

Helpful Tips for Relieving Vulvar Pain

1. A&D™ Ointment for babies works great on irritated vulvar skin. Apply a small amount of A&D™ Ointment to the vulva as needed to protect the skin. A&D™ also works great for women who experience increased friction in the vulvar area with walking.

2. Calendula cream applied to the vulvar area will help soothe irritated skin. Use on another body part first to make sure you are not allergic to it.

Calendula is derived from a flower and is used to soothe skin inflammation. You can also use a calendula wash and soap, which is described later in this chapter.

3. Too many times my patients use over-the-counter anti-yeast treatments only to make the burning and irritation worst. Do not use over-the-counter creams, ointments and anti-yeast medications without consulting your care-giver first. Prescription medications like Diflucan™ can also get rid of yeast infections without irritation to the vulva-vaginal area.

4. To soothe vulvar burning, some women find relief by using witch hazel pads (TUCKS Pads) to areas of discomfort. These pads are also a lifesaver after giving birth.

5. Taking lukewarm to warm baths helps with vulvar itching and burning. Fill the bath tub with a few inches of lukewarm to warm water and add colloidal oatmeal such as Aveeno™ to help reduce itching. If the Aveeno™ doesn't help, then try adding 4 to 5 tablespoons of baking soda to the bath to soothe vulvar itching and irritation.

6. Use sitz baths to relieve burning and irritation. A sitz bath is a bath in which the hips and buttock are submerged. Usually a small basin is used and placed on top of the toilet. After childbirth, using a sitz bath with Epsom salt can really help reduce pain and prevent infections. You can also steep calendula flowers and add the calendula water to your bath as well.

7. Apply a cool compress for 10 to 15 minutes to the vulva to help decrease pain and irritation. This technique is great if you have had a recent flare-up or severe vulvar pain.

Common Treatments for Perineal Vulvar Health

The perineum is an extremely sensitive area of the vulvar region that often undergoes trauma, especially during childbirth, when women may experience perineal tearing and episiotomies. Sometimes these wounds do not heal properly or do not heal at all, and continue to open up with intercourse, defecation and exercise. For persistent perineal wounds that do not seem to heal properly, work with your doctor or caregiver to find the right combination of medicines and vitamins that will complement your perineal stretching and scar mobilizations that I've outlined in Part III. The following is a list of remedies that my patients have tried with positive results, but make sure to work with your doctor to be certain of the combination that is right for your specific needs.

Vitamins to Improve Skin Conditions of the Perineum

To be taken internally and under the supervision a healthcare professional

1. Vitamin C
2. Vitamin A
3. Vitamin D
4. Vitamin E

Alternative Massage Oils and Creams for the Perineum

1. Vitamin E oil – Organic if possible
2. Rose oil and "Down There Oil" (see appendix)
3. Wild yam cream
4. Sesame Oil
5. Yoni cream
6. Calendula cream

Doctor-Prescribed Topical Creams and Medicines for the Perineum

1. Estrogen/Lidocaine combo

2. Testosterone cream

3. Estrogen/testosterone combo

4. Lidocaine

5. Steroidal cream

6. Elavil™

7. Muscle relaxers

8. Valium™ (suppositories can be used rectally or vaginally)

9. Estrogen E-ring for dryness of vagina, called atrophic vaginitis

10. Vagifem

11. Botox - internal injection

Vulvar Care and Clothing

1. Avoid wearing pantyhose. Use thigh or knee-high hose instead. If you must wear pantyhose, cut the crotch out.

2. Double rinse any clothes that come in contact with the vulva. Wash clothes with organic detergents. Avoid fabric softeners and dryer sheets on all clothing that comes in contact with the vulvar area. Whenever possible use organic, fragrance-free detergents.

3. Remove wet clothing immediately, especially after swimming and wash the vulvar area with water as soon as possible to avoid burning and inflammation that many times comes with swimming in a chlorinated pool.

4. Avoid wearing very tight jeans and pants and clothes made from synthetic fabrics that capture sweat and increase irritation. Also avoid low-rider jeans that can put pressure on the bladder area. Instead choose a pair of jeans that are loose and baggy in the crotch area of the pants and are loose around the waist.

5. Try wearing 100 percent cotton underwear. Many of my patients find that thongs increase vulvar irritation and many times also irritate the anal area.

Managing Vulvar Pain after Sexual Intercourse

1. Use water-soluble lubricants for sexual intercourse. When possible, use only organic products.

2. Urinate after sex.

3. Rinse the vulva with cool water after sex.

4. Apply a cold compress to the vulva immediately after sex to reduce irritation. Apply compress for at least 15 to 20 minutes for better results. Repeat every hour as necessary.

5. Lidocaine, commonly prescribed by doctors, helps reduce pain during sex. Lidocaine can sometimes burn for 3 to 5 minutes after application.

6. Focus on outercourse or tantric sex instead of intercourse when you are in pain. Experiment with lap dancing, oral sex, massage, mutual masturbation. Old-fashioned kissing can go a long way when you cannot have sexual intercourse.

7. If you are having intercourse, make sure you are both fully aroused and well-lubricated to reduce the actual penetration time and pain.

8. Make sure to do reverse Kegels before sexual penetration to reduce pain. Too many times my patients contract their muscles out of fear or habit right before intercourse, which increases their pain.

9. Experiment with different sexual positions to see which ones are the least painful.

10. Perform manual stretching with your finger or dilator before and after sex as highlighted in Part III of this book. This will allow the muscles to be more supple and relaxed.

Exercise and Vulvar Care

1. Avoid exercise that puts direct pressure on the vulva, such as biking and horseback riding. If you must bike, use padded pants and a padded seat or a bike seat designed to alleviate pressure on the pelvis such as the BiSaddle™, which has two mini seats built into one. Also try to limit the length of time you spend biking in general.

2. Low-impact exercises such as walking are great because they don't create a lot of friction in the vaginal area. For some, walking is not enough for them to really get their hearts pumping. High-impact exercises are acceptable as long as they don't increase your vulvar or vaginal discomfort. The best advice is to find cardiovascular exercises that don't increase gluteal, hip, or low-back muscle spasms, and especially vaginal pain. Cardiovascular exercise is important to do on a daily basis as it helps decrease stress, elevate natural endorphin levels (natural pain killers), and keep the heart and mind healthy. However, you have to find a balance so you don't worsen any painful symptoms.

3. Avoid exercising in highly synthetic materials that do not breathe and instead capture sweat. These types of materials increase vulvar irritation. Use cotton materials. Wear loose-fitting clothes and change your underwear immediately after exercise.

4. Perform the techniques in this book on a daily basis, especially the PFM stretching which will help reduce your pelvic pain.

5. Use a cool pack or ice pack on the vulva after exercising if pain increases. Wrap the cool pack up with 1 to 3 towels so that you don't cause damage to this very gentle skin. Cool packs and ice packs can be left on for 15 to 20 minutes.

6. Avoid classes like spinning and kickboxing which can throw out your hip and sacral alignment and put excessive pressure on the perineum. Practice your reverse Kegels as instructed in Part II so you can maintain your focus on your pelvic floor as you do your exercises.

Vaginal Steams for Vulvar/Vaginal Health and to Decrease Pain

Many of my patients swear by their vaginal steams and get great results with them. They experience less pain with sitting, have easier penetration, and are able to perform their vaginal stretches and insert dilators with more ease. I recommend doing vaginal steams on a weekly basis and even more often during painful flare-ups. Vaginal steams heat the pelvic floor muscles and help reduce tightness and muscle spasms. Vaginal steams should be avoided during your menstrual period or during pregnancy.

I recently treated a woman with a 10-year history of vaginismus. She had graduated to the largest dilator after several months of therapy, but was still experiencing pain and difficulty with its insertion. I recommended that she do a vaginal steam right before her dilator work. The following week she came to my office and was joyous. After her vaginal steam, she was able to insert the largest dilator without any problems. She said, "The dilator went right in, and I also had so much less pain with insertion."

Vaginal steams were taught to me by Dr. Rosita Arvigo, naturopathic doctor, renowned herbalist and Mayan healer. She has brought Maya Abdominal Massage to the United States and runs a great advanced certification program in Belize which I've completed. I find that many of the techniques of the Maya massage are essential for pelvic pain sufferers. The Arvigo Maya Abdominal Massage™ helps to realign the pelvic organs and decreases pelvic congestion by bringing healing energy and blood flow to the pelvic organs and pelvic floor muscles. With vaginal steams, you can mix and match the herbs and flowers you use depending on your condition. Consult a local herbalist before attempting to do a steam with herbs. Start your search on the web by checking out *www.ArvigoMassage.com*. You can also just start out with plain steamed water for the vaginal steams and still get results.

Vaginal Steam Instructions

1. Boil a gallon of water for 10 minutes and then let it steep with the herbs for 5 minutes with the lid on the pot.

2. Place water under a chair with open slits, or better yet place the bowl with the herbs into the toilet. Don't pour the steam solution into the toilet. Instead, put the whole pot into the toilet. Be careful as it might be too hot when you sit. If it feels too hot, you can also buy a raised toilet seat to avoid burns from the steam to the vulvar area/PFM.

3. Sit on the toilet and let the steam penetrate the PFMs via the vagina. If the steam is too hot, stand up and wait for it to cool down before sitting down again.

4. Wrap yourself in a blanket, put on socks, and make sure to avoid drafts while you are doing the steam. Sit down until all the steam has evaporated, about 15 to 20 minutes.

5. While sitting on the toilet, perform a reverse Kegel so that the pelvic

muscles are evenly heated and relaxed. The steam introduces heat into the pelvic muscles, helping them to relax and reduce spasms of the pelvic floor muscles.

6. Add to your vaginal steam water a mixture of dry flower and herbs. Dr. Arvigo has made a wonderful healing remedy for vaginal steams, using herbs and flowers like basil, oregano, calendula flowers and lavender.

7. After the vaginal steam, massage the vaginal muscles. This is also a great time to insert your dilator and rest in bed under warm sheets. Do your best after a steam to keep your body at a constant warm temperature for 24 hours, avoiding sudden drafts that might give you a chill.

8. Work with a local herbalist to see which flower/herb mixture might be the best for the specifics of your condition. See the following table for herbs and their uses. You will need one quart of the herbs if you are using fresh herbs and one cup if using dry herbs.

Table 12.1: Herbs That Can Be Used in Your Vaginal Steams

Note: This list is for educational purposes only. You must consult your physician or herbalist before using any of these herbs in a vaginal steam. These herbs should not be taken by pregnant and lactating women unless prescribed by your caregiver. The information in this table comes from www.mountainroseherbs.com.

NAME OF HERB	USES
Calendula	Helps to reduce pain naturally. Its antibacterial, antinflammatory, antifungal, and immunostimulant properties help treat slow-healing cuts. It soothes irritated, burning skin and also helps to stimulate collagen synthesis.
Basil	Helps restore immune function deficiency caused by stress. It also has antibacterial properties and helps other herbs penetrate the skin.

NAME OF HERB	USES
Motherwort	Helps with menstrual tension by acting as a uterine tonic. This herb has antibacterial, antifungal, antispasmodic, antiviral, and antiseptic properties.
Oregano	This herb has antispasmodic, antiviral, and antiseptic properties.
Rosemary	Has antioxidant, antiseptic, and antispasmodic properties. Helps to stop yeast from growing and helps to remove yeast cells from the urinary tract. Stimulates menstrual flow. Avoid this herb if your flow is already heavy.
St. John's Wort	Helps relieve pain. Should not be used together with Monoamine Oxidase Inhibitors (MAOIs) or Protease Inhibitors(PIs). Also helps to slow down frequent urination, and can treat throbbing pain of any origin.
Chamomile	Helps stop spasms in the smooth muscles and contains anti-inflammatory, antibacterial, antiviral, and antiparasitic properties.
Red Clover	Helps reduce pain associated with menstrual periods. Helps promote healing of skin wounds and reduces the effects of PMS and menopause. Avoid this herb if you are taking a blood thinner.
Marshmallow Root	Relieves irritation by coating inflamed surfaces; relieves vulva, perineal, and vestibular inflammation.

Daily Warm Baths to Relieve Muscle Spasms

One of the key recommendations that I make to my patients suffering from vaginal and PFM pain is warm baths. Not only do warm baths help reduce muscle spasms, but they also help reduce stress and anxiety. I recommend two baths a day, one before work and another at the end of the day right before going to bed. Make sure the bath water is not too hot and fill the tub so that your abdominals are entirely covered by the water. You may have to make the water less hot if you are having vulvar skin irritation. If tolerated, try adding Epsom salt or sea salt to the bath water. These salts help relax the muscles and thereby help to lower your pain naturally.

Calendula Wash

WHAT TO DO:

1. Boil a handful of calendula in 2 cups of water.

2. Let the mixture stand for 30 minutes or until the water turns amber.

3. Wait until the solution is room temperature, then add to your tub or sitz bath. If possible, sit for 30 minutes in your calendula bath.

4. During the immediate post-partum period, put the calendula wash into a perineal spritz bottle and use it to rinse the vulva after urination.

Ice/Heat Packs

Ice Packs or Cool Packs: These are great to use after sex if there's a lot of burning and irritation. Make sure you wrap the ice pack in a towel or T-shirt to avoid burns. Use for 10 to 20 minutes or as needed.

Traditional Hot Packs: I always recommend moist heat or hot water bottles but an electric pad would do as well. Make sure to wrap the hot packs to avoid burning yourself. Place the hot pack for 10 to15 minutes and repeat the application as needed. There are many places you can place the packs; it all depends on where the pain is. The following is a list of places that are usually affected by pelvic pain and benefit from heat. You can also try ice and see what works better for you.

1. Vulva (make sure the heat source is wrapped in a towel or T-shirt)
2. Inner thighs
3. Gluteal muscles
4. Lower back, tailbone or sacroiliac joint area
5. Between gluteal muscles on the rectal area
6. Abdominal muscles (great to apply before abdominal rolling)

Portable Cold/Hot Packs: Many of my patients find relief with their hot or cold packs. It always surprises me that such a simple modality can have dramatic effects in reducing pelvic pain and muscle spasms. My patients also love their portable heat and ice pads. These pads can bring comfort and help reduce pain while you are at work or during long plane trips, and can be used everyday to help keep painful muscle spasms at bay. They can be purchased at any pharmacy and are light and easy to put in your purse. Always follow the directions for your portable cold and hot packs.

Castor Oil Packs

Castor oil has been used for medicinal purposes dating back to ancient Egypt. It is derived from the bean of the ricinus communis plant also called palma christi because of its palm-shaped leaves and its miraculous healing properties. Castor oil packs were introduced by Edgar Cayce, the father of modern holistic medicine. Castor oil packs are the external use of castor oil and are commonly used by alternative healers for a variety of conditions and health problems.

Castor oil packs help to promote healing of the tissues and organs underneath the skin. They help increase blood and lymphatic flow, relieve constipation and decrease congestion of abdominal organs. Additionally castor oil packs can improve the autoimmune system, relieve pain from arthritis and tendonitis, and are used to break up scar and abdominal adhesions. For pelvic-pain patients castor oil packs are commonly used to decrease pelvic congestion by improving blood circulation to the abdominal organs. Many women use castor oil packs to break up adhesions after abdominal surgeries. Others use the packs to treat fibroids, ovarian cysts and to improve fertility.

WHAT TO DO:

1. Soak flannel or cotton material in castor oil so that it is thoroughly soaked and saturated but not dripping wet.

2. Place the pack over the affected body part. Cover the castor oil with plastic. Place the hot water bottle or heating pad over the pack. When using a heating pad put in on the medium to high setting. **Do not fall asleep with the heating pad on. Make sure to use a heating pad with an automatic shut-off button.**

3. Leave it on for 45 to 60 minutes. Rest while the pack is in place. This is a great time to meditate and/or practice your reverse Kegels.

4. It is generally recommended for non-acute conditions to use a castor oil pack 3 times per week, every other day. On the fourth week, rest and do not apply a castor oil pack. It is best to consult with your healthcare provider for your specific treatment regimen.

5. After removing the pack, cleanse your skin with a diluted solution of water and baking soda.

6. Store the pack in a covered container in the refrigerator. Each pack may be reused up to 25 to 30 times and can last for 6 months.

WHAT TO WATCH OUT FOR:

1. Castor oil should not be taken internally, as it is a harsh laxative.

2. Castor oil packs should not be applied to broken skin.

3. Castor oil should not be used on C-section or abdominal scars before 6 weeks. Please make sure to consult your doctor before applying a castor oil pack to your scars.

4. Castor oil packs should not be used during pregnancy, breastfeeding, or during menstrual flow.

Chapter Thirteen

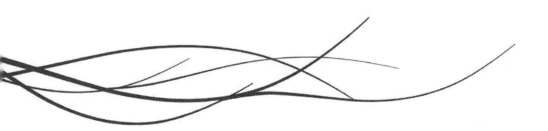

"Forgiveness is the fragrance the violet
sheds on the heel that has crushed it."
— Mark Twain

Chapter 13

BETTER BATHROOM HABITS

As unbelievable as it sounds, something as simple as bad bathroom habits compounded over many years can often be the root cause of pelvic pain and muscle spasms. Many of my patients are surprised to hear that they have been going to the bathroom incorrectly for years and are even more surprised at how much relief they get once they make a few corrections to their basic voiding habits. Oftentimes people are not aware or do not focus their attention when they are in the bathroom, and the results can be prolonged painful flare-ups and overall vulvar irritation. Proper potty posture is one of the simplest and most effective techniques in your toolbox that will have a tremendous impact on your overall healing journey.

Proper Potty Posture

1. Sit with knees above hips, legs wide apart and feet plantar flexed, which means on your toes. For women under five feet tall, use a footstool or book if necessary. Taller women may not need to elevate feet to maintain the above position.

2. Lean forward and place elbows on your thighs. Keep the arch in your back and avoid slumping or rounding the lower back.

3. Gently bulge out your abdominals while simultaneously widening your waist as if to "brace" yourself from a blow to the abdomen.

4. Once you can bulge and brace simultaneously this can be used as a toilet technique, as it will help relax the pelvic floor muscles and facilitate defecation. Doing the "potty posture" takes time but with practice you will master it.

5. Avoid straining. Do not hold your breath. Instead, grunt or groan while bearing down. Play with different sounds such as *ooh*, *ah*, and *shh* which will help further relax your pelvic floor muscles.

Top Bathroom Habits

1. Avoid Constipation. Most individuals who suffer from constipation push and strain to get the stool out. This excessive straining adversely affects your pelvic floor muscles, causing them to be more stressed, leading to increased muscle spasms and pain. **Strategy:** Make sure to get an adequate amount of fiber, drink plenty of water, and always use the "potty posture" as described in the earlier pages of this chapter.

2. Avoid Pushing Urine Out. Most of my patients who suffer from pelvic pain and pelvic floor muscle tightness always complain that they feel as though they can't get the urine out (called feelings of incomplete emptying) or that it takes awhile for the urine stream to start (called hesitancy of urine flow). This makes them push to get the urine out. As stated before, pushing or forcing urination leads to pelvic floor muscle strain which eventually will increase your pelvic pain. **Strategy:** If you are having trouble getting the urine out without pushing, perform quick Kegels and then return to the bathroom later, or try getting up from the toilet, standing for a few minutes, and then sit down again.

3. Avoid Poor Potty Posture. Avoid poor body mechanics and postural alignment such as rounded lower back or slumped upper back while seated on the toilet during defecation. **Strategy:** Use correct "potty posture" to align your spine and internal organs and relax your pelvic floor muscles. This will facilitate elimination without strain or stress on the pelvic floor muscles. Also, remember to never hold your breath with defecation or elimination as this will stress your pelvic floor muscles.

4. Avoid Poor Bladder Health and Habits. Avoid urinating out of habit instead of when a proper urge is present to maintain excellent bladder health. **Strategy:** Normal voiding is 6 to 8 times a day, with a 4 to 5 hour

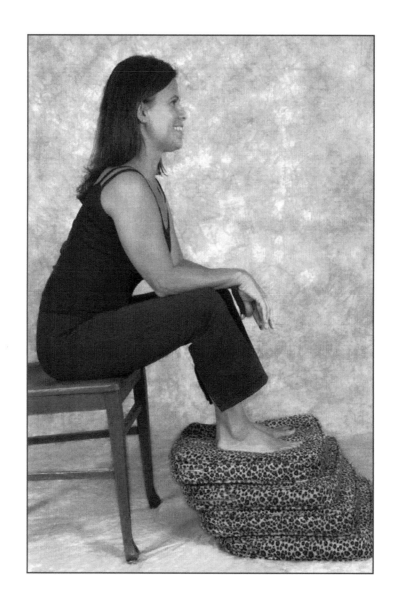

interval. If you do not meet the above criteria, get help in establishing better bladder health. Ask your physical therapist, urologist, internist, or other caregiver to help you get on the right track. Make sure you are also taking in enough water to avoid having highly concentrated urine, a bladder irritant which contributes to an increased urge to urinate.

Tracking Your Bladder and Bowel Health

To bring awareness and to start normalizing your bladder and bowel health, keep track of your voiding and defecation. I have included a voiding diary in Table 13.1 that you can use for tracking your habits as you begin to correct issues that you may not even be aware are contributing to your condition. Once you have filled in your diary, take it to your physical therapist, urologist, or nurse and let them help you reestablish proper habits. In the following chart, ask yourself the following:

1. What is your voiding interval? Is it 15 minutes, 45 minutes, 4 hours, etc?

2. What foods are you eating that could be causing bladder irritation? For a complete guide to foods that cause bladder irritation, consult the fantastic online resource at *www.ic-network.com*.

3. Do you feel like you have to urinate all the time (urgency of urination)? If so, use the following urge-suppression techniques.

    a. Distraction of the mind to delay voiding

    b. Quick-flick Kegels, as covered in Part II on page 75.

    c. Diaphragmatic breathing

4. How much water are you drinking during the day? Drink at least 6 to 8 cups of water per day to keep urine diluted. Concentrated urine is highly irritating to the bladder.

Table 13.1: Daily Voiding Diary

PDF version of this table available at http://www.RenewPT.com

Time of Day	Food Intake	Water Intake (ounces)	Amount Urinated (counted in Mississippis)	Urge Present or Leaking? (Y/N)
6AM				
7AM				
8AM				
9AM				
10AM				
11AM				
12PM				
1PM				
2PM				
3PM				
4PM				
5PM				
6PM				
7PM				
8PM				
9PM				
10PM				
11PM				
12AM				
Overnight				

Chapter Fourteen

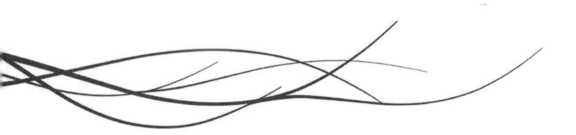

"Most of the important things in the world have been accomplished by people who have kept on trying when there seemed to be no hope at all."
- Dale Carnegie

Chapter 14

TRICKS OF THE TRADE

In order to fight back and take control of your pain, you need to have at your disposal a vast arsenal of tools. You could always just take lots of Motrin™ or stronger pain medications to control pain and numb the mind, but at the end of the day these just mask the root causes of pain. My goal is for you to have the tools and food for thought that will help you regain your inner peace, eliminate pain, and give you a better long-term approach for future flare-ups or moments when your pain may reoccur. Some of the techniques in this chapter describe how to use tools that are readily available, such as tennis balls, Thera Canes™, and Knobbles™. Other techniques I want you to have in your toolkit include electrical stimulation (TENS) and biofeedback technology, both of which you would have to consult your physical therapist or doctor to obtain. I have also included a detailed description of some effective strain-counterstrain techniques that you can do yourself, which are fantastic techniques for releasing spasms and pain in the muscles of your pelvic floor and the muscles that are in close relationship to the PFMs. If you incorporate these trade secrets into your self-healing journey, you can improve your chances of obtaining long-lasting pain relief.

Tennis Ball Massage for Piriformis Release

My patients swear by their tennis balls for pain relief in the lower back and gluteal areas. What I recommend is that they place a tennis ball on the painful body parts and roll it back and forth until the pain starts to dissipate. At first the pain can be excruciating but the longer you do it the better you will feel. Experiment with what works best for you. Sometimes I have my patients just keep the

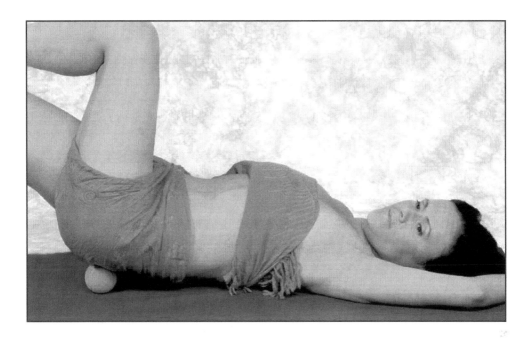

tennis ball stationary on the most painful spot of most pain for 60 to 90 seconds and then have them begin to roll the ball around the painful area. With consistency the result is almost always a reduction in pain and a loosening of painful trigger points.

Common locations for Tennis Ball Massage:

1. Gluteal muscles

2. Upper hip muscles

3. Upper back muscles

4. Sacrum

5. Hip bones

6. On either side of the spine, you can use two tennis balls simultaneously.

Thera Cane™

The Thera Cane™ is a great tool for trigger point releases in painful muscles and works great on muscles that are difficult to reach. Place the Thera Cane™ on the painful spot and hold it against the area with consistent pressure for 60 to 90 seconds. Repeat as needed. One of the best resources on the market for the use of the Thera Cane™ is *The Trigger Point Therapy Workbook* by Claire Davies.

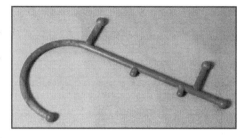

Theracane™

Recommended areas for Thera Cane™ placement:

1. Inner thigh muscles

2. Gluteal muscles

3. Lower back muscles including the quadratus lumborum

4. Upper back

5. Abdominal muscles, avoiding artery pulses in the abdominal muscles

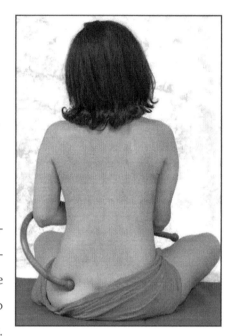

Psoas Release with Thera Cane™

Your body has 2 very deep muscles on either side of the lower abdomen called the psoas muscles. These muscles attach from the lower spine to the hip bones, and help flex the hips. The psoas muscles are frequently very painful, in spasm, and irritated in females suffering from pelvic pain.

To find the psoas muscles do the following:

1. Lie on your back with your legs straight out.

2. Go about 2 to 3 inches to the right side of your belly button. Place your fingertips into the area, slowly allowing them to sink into your abdomen and being careful to avoid any feelings of an artery pulse.

3. Lift your right leg straight up and you will feel the psoas pop into your hand. It may take a little practice to get this down but keep trying. Now that you know where the psoas muscle is, place your Thera Cane™ in that spot and slowly press downward into the psoas for 60 to 90 seconds. If you feel any tingling, numbness, or tremendous increase in pain, get off the area and try to relocate the psoas muscle. Switch sides and do the left psoas muscle release.

The Knobble™

The Knobble™ is a smaller version of the Thera Cane™ and is a great tool to use on trigger points. For best results, find the painful spots and press the Knobble™ into the spot for 60 to 90 seconds. The great thing about the Knobble™ is that it easily fits into you purse and can be taken with you to work or when you are away from home on vacation.

Common Areas for the Knobble:

1. Inner thigh
2. Abdominals
3. Gluteal muscles
4. Psoas muscle
5. Low back muscles
6. Upper hip muscles

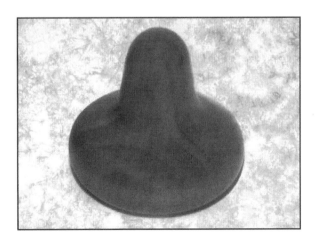

TENS Unit

Transcutaneous Electrical Stimulation (TENS) is a noninvasive, nonaddictive, drug-free tool that helps many of my patients manage their pelvic pain. You will have to get a prescription from your doctor to get a TENS unit. Prices range from $50 to $1000, so shop wisely. Many times insurance will cover the cost of the units.

How Does It Work?

Soft conductive pads transmit low voltage electrical impulses to areas where the pads are placed. These electrical impulses suppress pain by blocking pain signals before they reach the brain. Pain relief varies among individuals. For some, pain relief is felt immediately while the TENS unit is on. For others, relief continues even after the unit is turned off.

Wearing a TENS unit can bring relief while doing your daily activities. Many of my patients wear a smaller-sized TENS units that can be clipped on their clothes while at work or traveling long distances.

Finding the right placement and setting for your TENS unit is key in reducing pelvic, bladder and lower back pain. Work with your physical therapist to find the right energy pulse setting depending on the exact nature of your condition. Your therapist can also help you with the correct placement of the pads. The large electrodes allow a lot of area to be covered so pad placement does not have to be exact. In the next few pages you will see my most tried and true TENS pad placements that give you relief.

Location of Pads of the TENS Unit

See photos for correct electrode placement.

1. **Along the spine** to the side of pain.

Helps reduce low back pain, hip pain, and general pelvic pain.

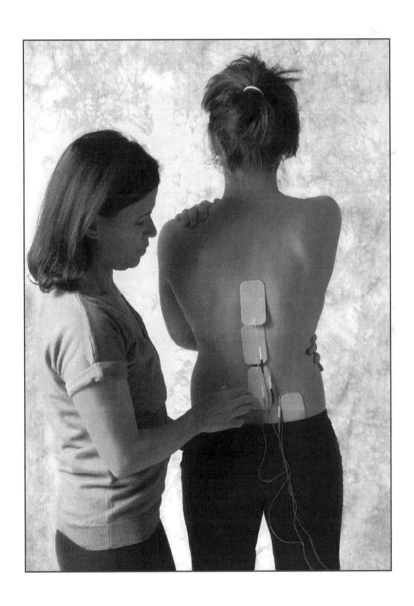

2. **Lower back**

Helps reduce sacral pain, low back pain, hip pain, and pelvic pain. Pads go on either side of the spine in the low back area.

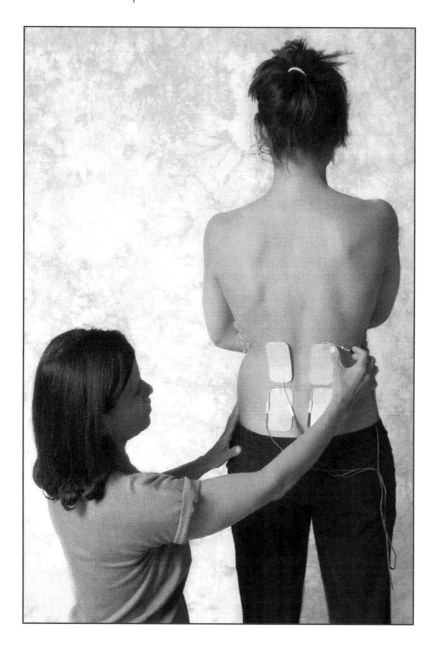

3. Lower back and gluteal muscles

Helps reduce low back, pelvic, and gluteal pain, and sciatica.

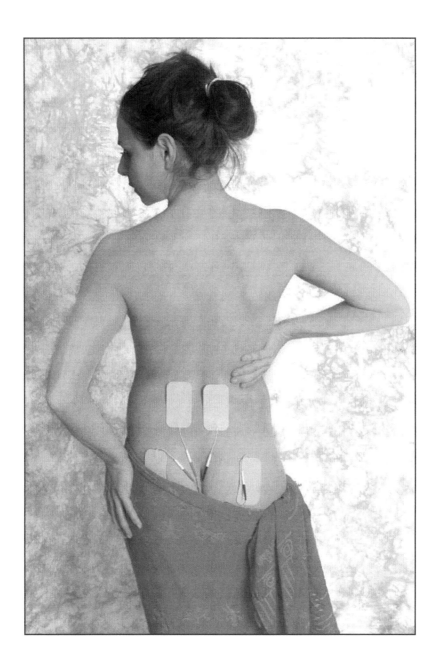

4. **Pudendal nerve**

Helps reduce pain with pudendal nerve neuropathy and pain with sitting.

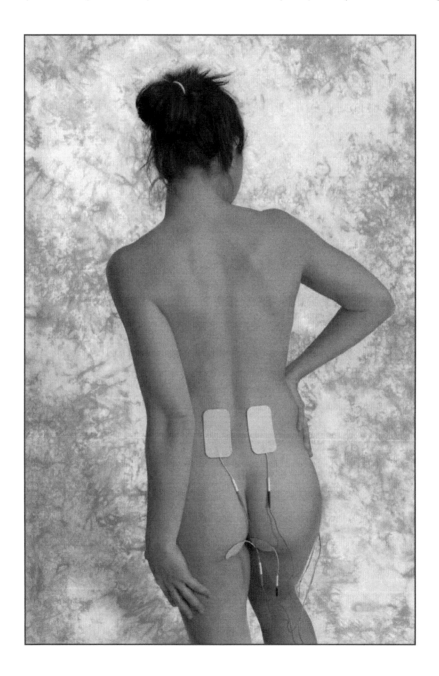

5. **Bladder**

Helps reduce pain with sitting, pain with positional changes, bladder pain, and generalized pelvic pain. Place pads in a semicircle near and around pubic and hip bones.

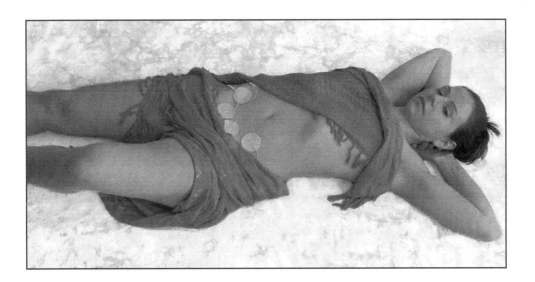

Biofeedback Technology

Biofeedback technology is a great tool for pelvic floor muscle retraining because it allows you to visualize your PFMs, which are difficult to see. I use biofeedback in conjunction with the various techniques listed throughout this book because it gives me an objective measure and helps me establish a treatment plan for my patient. Biofeedback uses sensors, both externally and/or internally to get electrical readouts from the muscles and how they perform. The units I use in the healing center hook up to a laptop and provide great visuals for my patients so they can see when they are doing Kegels correctly, or downtraining their PFMs correctly. Once they see the readout and feel how the PFMs should be working, it is much easier to repeat the techniques and exercises at home.

The biofeedback also gives me a reading of a patient's resting baseline measured in microvolts, so I can know if their "relaxed state" is truly relaxed.

Usually a pelvic pain patient will have a high resting baseline with the biofeedback of over 2 microvolts. Biofeedback is scientific and allows the patient to understand what it feels like to relax and to let go of the tension in these muscles as they try to lower their baseline.

Biofeedback training might be covered by your health insurance plan. I recommend doing biofeedback with guidance of a physical therapist that can help to cue you. Some facilities do what is called unguided biofeedback, where you are left alone in the room to figure things out for yourself, which I do not recommend. Once you get the basics down with your physical therapist, you can also rent these machines and reeducate your muscles in the privacy of your own home.

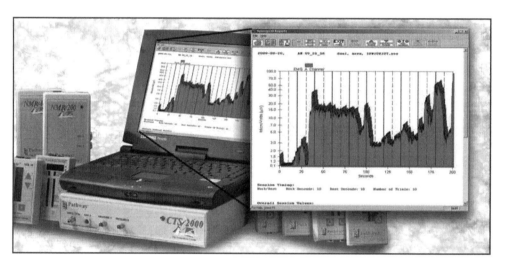

Biofeedback is a great way to get a readout of how your muscles are working together. Through internal and external sensors, the software provides your PFM muscle baseline output in microvolts, helping you visualize while downtraining or uptraining.

Strain-Counterstrain

Strain-counterstrain techniques can have dramatic pain-relieving effects for those suffering from pelvic, hip, and gluteal pain. I have found that when I use these techniques as part of my patients' treatment sessions they often get immediate relief, and have better mobility and improved range of motion in stubborn, tight muscles.

The strain-counterstrain technique was developed by Dr. Lawrence Jones, an osteopathic doctor. It is a gentle and safe technique that passively shortens the affected muscle areas by holding those muscles in a contracted state for 90 seconds. When the muscle is held in this position, it gradually returns to its original resting position and length and is therefore less painful. It's pretty easy to do as part of your self-care as well. These techniques are great to use with a partner but you can also just use them on your own with some modifications. I have included the top two that I think are the easiest to do on yourself and that could give you the most pain relief.

Always grade your pain on a scale of 0 to 10. Grading your pain this way tracks your progress to see if your pain is improving. Remember, it is important to come out of this position slowly and mindfully. Also keep in mind that strain-counterstrain techniques are great to use during your period as they are both external methods.

Obturator Internus Strain-Counterstrain

Obturator internus (OI) pain is very common in woman with vulvodynia. Frequently, pain with deep sexual thrusting can be a result of trigger points or spasms located in this muscle. This muscle is a big culprit of sexual pain as the pudendal nerve travels in its fascia and the pelvic floor muscles also have a connection to this muscle.

WHAT TO DO:

1. Lie on your stomach, find your right sit bone with your right hand and go slightly medial to it, towards the inside of the bone. Press inwards towards the right sit bone and look for painful spots. Here is where the trigger point is commonly found for the OI.

2. While holding the spot with your right hand, bend your right knee to 90 degrees and allow the foot to fall inwards, producing external rotation of the hip. The OI muscle will "pop" into your hand.

3. Hold the spot with the knee bent and rotated for 90 seconds and retest to see if your pain has decreased. Repeat on the left side.

General Pelvic Floor Muscle (Pubococcygeus and Iliococcygeus) Strain-Counterstrain

This strain-counterstrain alleviates overall pelvic floor muscle pain. Symptoms associated with dysfunction in the pelvic floor muscles could be pelvic pain, rectal pain, deep sexual thrusting pain, pubic bone pain, and bladder issues. It is very simple to do and a powerful technique for a generalized pelvic floor muscle release.

WHAT TO DO:

1. To locate this trigger point, palpate internally inside the vagina or find it in the perineum near the sit bones and coccyx/tailbone area.

2. Lie on your back with your hips and knees bent and place a towel under your sacrum and coccyx/tailbone area.

3. Place your right hand over your pubic bone and press the pubic bone with your fingers towards your back, and hold for 90 seconds.

Bulbospongiosus Strain-Counterstrain

The bulbospongiosus is part of the first layer of the pelvic floor muscles. If the bulbocavernosus muscle is in spasms or has trigger points in it there can be pain with initial sexual penetration. If this muscle is in extreme spasms, there might not be any penetration at all. This technique can be extremely helpful before sexual intercourse or as part of your dilator healing program.

WHAT TO DO:

1. Start comfortably in an inclined seated position propped up on some pillows. It's best to remove your underwear for this strain-counterstrain method.

2. Place your index and ring fingers on either side of the clitoris and press your fingers downward towards your perineal body.

3. Place another finger from your other hand over your perineal body and press the perineal body in a superior direction towards your clitoris. You're basically bringing both parts towards each other. Hold this shortened position for 90 seconds. Repeat as necessary.

Proprioceptive Neuromuscular Techniques (PNF)

PNF techniques, short for Proprioceptive Neuromuscular Facilitation isometric techniques, can help release tension in the pelvic floor muscles naturally. The following PNF pattern works particularly well to help maintain a relaxed state in the PFMs.

WHAT TO DO:

1. Lie on your back with your knees bent and aligned with your hips so that your hips and knees form a right angle.

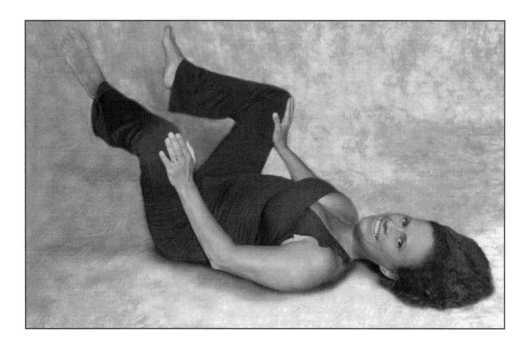

2. Place your hands on the top of your knees, allowing your knees to move outward, as in the photo.

3. As you exhale, press your hands into your knees and your knees into your hands, giving yourself resistance, but not allowing the position to change.

4. The line of force is going to be towards your shoulders, but don't let your hands or legs move.

5. Concentrate on feeling the relaxation of the PFMs and then try to perform a reverse Kegel.

6. Hold for 10 seconds, rest for 10 seconds, repeat 3 times per set, 2 to 3 times per day.

Let's tie it all together now by connecting our physical bodies to our minds by using the techniques in the next chapter, to end the mental chatter that actually contributes to the cycle of pain more than you can imagine.

Chapter Fifteen

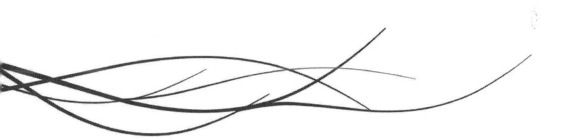

*"Adversity causes some men to break;
others to break records."*
– William Arthur Ward

Chapter 15

MIND/BODY VISUALIZATIONS
AND LIFE STRATEGY TECHNIQUES

Chronic pelvic pain can have devastating effects on a woman's life. The sense of loss and isolation that often accompanies this condition can leave a large hole in your heart and soul. The women that I treat come to their sessions with such sadness that it is difficult for them to hide the demoralizing effects that chronic pelvic pain has on their lives. Many of my patients tell me their partners end up leaving them because they are unable to participate fully in a sexual relationship, causing depression and pessimism to overtake their lives. Many others live in strained relationships with their partners. No matter how you see it, pelvic pain is a difficult condition to live with.

Typical Stories

My patient Harriet, who loved her man very much, couldn't have sex with him anymore because the pain was just too much to bear. In the end, Harriet's boyfriend left her because of the problems with intimacy. The bad part was that Harriet did not want to get involved in a relationship again, which I commonly see in my patients with chronic pain. She's lived her life in isolation and fear that she would never get better again. Every time she meets a man she gets nervous and stresses out because she knows the topic of sex will come up, and she's still not well enough to participate in a sexual relationship. Another patient Lynn, a beautiful young woman, got involved with a much older man because she knew he would not request sex from her. She seemed okay with the relationship but she told me she doesn't really love him. His companionship means a lot to her even if there was no sex, but she was left depressed and pessimistic.

There's also Michelle, a high-powered lawyer who worked so many hours she had "no time" for romance. The long hours kept her safely in a cocoon so she wouldn't have to put herself out there. The stress of Michelle's job would exacerbate her symptoms to the point that when she got home at night she would have to take a pain killer to sleep at night.

Another woman Danelle shows the great length that women will go to have a sexual relationship in spite of their chronic pelvic pain. After Danelle had her baby she could no longer have sex without pain. She experienced a third-degree perineal tear during birth and reported feeling that the attending doctor closed her vagina up too tightly, such that her husband now no longer fit into her vagina. She would try to satisfy her husband with oral stimulation, but eventually he became frustrated, angry and resentful because of the lack of sex. Danelle also felt trapped, depressed and became filled with pessimism, feeling that she did not have a choice because she didn't want a divorce.

As you can see in the previous examples, many of my patients who suffer from chronic pain experience an array of emotions that include hopelessness, despair, sadness and catastrophic thinking that contributes to their feelings that they will never get better. These feelings only get worse when the pain is compounded over the years, making them feel out of control. Suffering from chronic pelvic pain can rob you of precious life moments because the pain cycle does not always allow you to participate fully in relationships. Oftentimes, even jobs are affected since many chronic pain sufferers have to miss work.

What I have observed from patients is that if you don't address the mental component of your pain, your condition will create havoc on your mind, soul and body. Although chronic stress does not cause pelvic pain, chronic stress and pessimism can make the pain worse, making you more sensitive to pain and thus causing more flare-ups. I also find it very difficult to treat patients successfully when they are chronically negative and in a state of stress. Many times I have to get them to relax during their treatment sessions before we can even do any treatments. When I incorporate mind-body relaxation techniques into my patients' self-care and home exercise programs, they always do better in the long-term. What I have also noticed is that women who do the best with my treatments are those who are able to defeat negativity by incorporating stress reduction mind-body techniques as part of their healing program.

The Physiology of Stress

Your body undergoes many physiological changes when you become stressed out. The first thing that happens is that your endocrine system reacts by releasing many different types of stress hormones into your bloodstream including adrenaline and cortisol. These hormones awaken you mentally, physically and prepare your body for an emergency response. The body goes through physical changes as well, including increased heart rate, tightening of the muscles, increased sharpness and keenness of the five senses, elevation of blood pressure, increase in perspiration, and shunting of blood from the small muscles to the large muscles of the arms and legs. In addition, your physical strength increases, your reaction time gets faster, and your focus is sharper. These bodily changes prepare you to either fight or flee from a dangerous situation. When real danger is present, stress is a good thing and can motivate you to perform better in life. But when stress is an everyday occurrence it can be detrimental to your health and relationships, eventually clouding your thinking and leading to feelings of being overwhelmed. If you're stressed over a busy schedule, an argument with a friend, a traffic jam, or a mountain of bills, your body reacts just as strongly as if you were facing a life-or-death situation. If you have a lot of responsibilities and worries, your emergency stress response may be "on" most of the time. The more your body's stress system is activated, the easier it is to fall into a pain response or flare-up and the harder it is to shut it off.

Long-term stress can even rewire the brain, leaving you more vulnerable to anxiety and depression. Researchers at the Northwestern University Institute of Neuroscience found that people suffering with chronic back pain, for example, not only demonstrate abnormal brain chemistry, particularly in the emotional center of the brain, but also actual brain shrinkage (*The Journal of Neuroscience,* November, 2004).

For pelvic pain sufferers it is extremely important to manage stress and keep it in check. I have included several techniques and exercises that I use as part of my Renew Program for Women™, helping my patients manage their stress and overcome catastrophic thinking. These stress reduction techniques, meditations, affirmations, and visualizations are easy to do and require no special equipment and can be done anywhere and anytime.

Table15.1: Stress Reduction Techniques

Frequency: Daily

TECHNIQUE
1. Breathing
2. Cardiovascular Stress Reduction
3. Progressive Relaxation with Jacobson's Techniques
4. Positive Thinking vs. Negative Self-Talk
5. Mantras and Meditation
6. Journaling
7. Affirmations
8. Keep It Simple – Stop Taking on Too Much
9. Join a Self-Help Group
10. Gratitude Training – Rock and Walk
11. The Present Moment – Staying in the Power of Now
12. Creative Visualizations

Breathing

Focusing on your breathing can have tremendous benefits for your overall stress level. It also helps you to quiet your mind and centers your attention on the present moment. Most people don't take the time to focus on their breathing during the course of the day, but this powerful yet simple exercise can help you release tension, stress, and anxiety.

WHAT TO DO:

1. Sit in cross-legged position, stand or lie down in a relaxed comfortable position.

2. Slowly inhale through your nose, counting to 5 in your head.

3. Exhale from your mouth, counting to 10 in your head. The exhale counting depends on your comfort. Some women may find that exhaling for 10 seconds is too long and causes anxiety or shortness of breath.

TIPS:

1. As you breathe, let your lower abdomen expand outward, keeping your shoulders quiet and low. Avoid raising your shoulders as you inhale and exhale. Breathing this way enhances relaxation and it's a natural way to breathe. Breathing like this also helps fill your lungs more fully with fresh air and helps to release old stagnant air.

2. Repeat several times a day for 5 to 10 minutes. Great to do at work, during stressful situations, and while meditating.

3. To release more tension, exhale so the air comes out like a whisper by pursing lips. This kind of breathing is done in many yoga classes.

4. Focus on releasing your stress in your exhale, attaching your stress to your breath as it leaves your body.

Cardiovascular Stress Reduction

Cardiovascular exercise for at least 30 minutes a day is a great stress buster and it also helps to release natural endorphins that help relieve pain. The one exercise that anyone can do is walking which is why I always recommend a walking program to release stress.

WHAT TO DO:

1. Walk during your lunch hour instead of having lunch at your desk. Follow your lunch-time walk with the workplace stretches listed in Chapter 7 of this book.

2. Take an evening walk after dinner instead of sitting in front of your computer or sitting to watch TV.

3. Join a gym and walk on the treadmill when it's cold outside. You can also do a walking program in a mall when it's cold outside.

4. Combine your walking with your gratitude meditation as well, which I will describe later in this chapter. This is a really positive way to build a permanent change to your overall thought patterns.

5. As an alternative to walking, try stationary biking and then see how you feel. Make sure you wear padded bike pants. Be careful of the bikes, though, because they can add too much pressure on the perineum and pelvic floor muscles.

Progressive Relaxation with Jacobson's Techniques

Progressive muscle relaxation was developed by Dr. Edmund Jacobson more than 50 years ago. Dr. Jacobson discovered through his work with his patients that a muscle could be relaxed by first voluntarily tensing it for a few seconds. This voluntary contraction and subsequent muscle relaxation of various body areas produces a deep state of relaxation. Dr. Jacobson found that this technique of progressive relaxation was capable of relieving a variety of conditions, from high blood pressure to ulcerative colitis, to overall pain.

GENERAL GUIDELINES:

This relaxation technique requires that you alternately tense and relax your muscles. Try to practice this relaxation at the same time each day for 15 to 30 minutes. Find a comfortable position such as supported incline sitting or lying down. Start with the breathing techniques described above for 5 to 10 minutes. The best way to start is to work with groups of muscles in the following sequence but you can also develop a system that works for you.

Basic Jacobson Contract/Relax Sequence

WHAT TO DO:

1. Contract the right arm for 10 seconds and then relax your right arm for 15 to 20 seconds. Do the same for left arm.

2. Contract both shoulders for 10 seconds and then relax your shoulders for 15 to 20 seconds.

3. Contract your neck muscles for 10 seconds and then relax your neck muscles for 15 to 20 seconds.

4. Contract your lips and eyes by closing them tightly for 10 seconds and then relax your lips and eyes for 15 to 20 seconds.

5. Contract whole right leg including toes and ankle tightly for 10 seconds and then relax your whole right leg for 15 to 20 seconds. Do the same for the left leg.

6. This is a basic sequence but you can separate out the body parts and tense and relax as many body parts as you want. The more body parts you individually contract and relax the longer this relaxation will take.

Positive Thinking vs. Negative Self-Talk

Oftentimes, my patients can be their own worst enemies. Self-sabotaging thoughts in the form of negative self-talk prevent them from doing the things they need to do to get better. Sometimes the self-sabotaging thoughts are even subconscious, and my patients don't even realize they are doing it habitually until I point it out to them. These women are filled with thoughts such as "I'll never get better," "sex will always hurt," and "this is the best I will ever feel."

I am a firm believer that the body will follow your mind. What you think is what you are. The way we talk to ourselves can make a situation sunny and bright or can take the same situation and make it dark, cloudy and gloomy. Pay attention to the story that your thoughts are creating about your life. Acknowledge your thoughts, but don't always take them as gospel. You can change your entire life by first changing your negative self-talk into more positive, focused and optimistic thought patterns.

Mantras and Meditation

I give my patients mantras to get them through the day. A mantra is a repeated word, syllable, phrase, or sound that can help you relax during times of stress or as a precursor to your stretching, strengthening or dilator work. Saying a mantra during meditation or at various times throughout the day will help quiet your mind and bring inner peace to you. The most basic mantra is OM. This mantra can be repeated slowly for 3 to 5 minutes and it brings a calming feeling to your entire body. Allow the syllable or syllables of your mantra to resonate slowly inside your head and body like a bell, using it to clear out the "thought clutter" that often prevents us from staying in the moment. The main objective is to quiet down negative thoughts to make room for positive thoughts to sprout into your consciousness. Remember, you must believe in your mantra, and then your body will follow. I like to have my patients meditate for 3 to 5 minutes while quietly repeating their mantra. This meditation technique with mantras has been shown to lower cholesterol, reduce stress, pain, and blood pressure, and improve heart function.

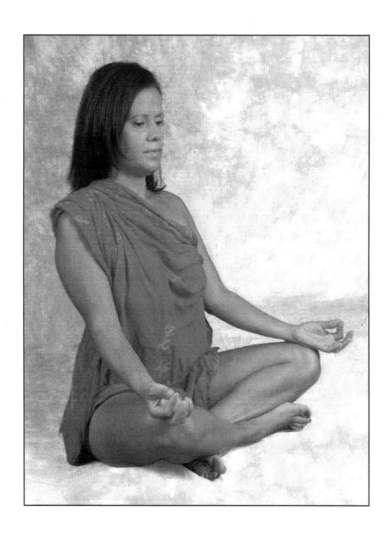

WHAT TO DO:

1. Sit or lie down, usually with your eyes closed.

2. Focus on deep diaphragmatic breathing for 5 to 10 breaths as you slow down your mind. Many of my patients report holding their breath or breathing shallowly when they experience pain, which limits oxygen to the tissues and results in more pain. You must do the opposite during your meditation.

3. Begin repeating your mantra with conviction, allowing it to permeate into your being.

4. After 3 to 5 minutes, resume diaphragmatic breathing and then after you feel comfortable, repeat the mantra or try a different one.

Mantra Samples

Om Shanti Om

I-Am-Pain-Free

I-Am-Healed

Journaling

I often tell my patients to keep a journal of their journeys up to the present moment. I tell them to write down the stories of their pain as they perceive it. Sometimes the pain is a result of a traumatic incident from childhood. I had a patient tell me she had her pain since she fell off a trampoline as a youngster. Other patients don't tell me but I get a sense that their pain is the result of sexual abuse. Oftentimes they don't completely remember what happened but they feel that their body's response has been one of "closing down" in an effort to protect itself. Still other patients' pain journeys are the result of giving birth to their children and not getting the proper care and encouragement to get their bodies back. Other new moms carry a sense of shame because they had

C-sections instead of natural births, and thus develop pain as it relates to their low self-esteem surrounding their birth experience.

Whatever the story of your pain may be, I encourage my patients to write it down and track their feelings as they journey forward with The Renew Program for Women™. Once you have it written down, I often suggest my patients to perform a ceremony where they burn or shred their story and release the past from their body and mind. I first did this after a painful, late-stage miscarriage. My husband and I were filled with pain and anguish, and thought we could not move forward. We ended up journeying to the mountains in Spain where we burned the printouts of the sonograms of our baby, releasing the past from our psyches. It was hard to do but it ended up being a wonderful experience that brought us tremendous feelings of peace and acceptance, and cleared out the past. Once you let go of the mental burden of your own pain story, you can free your consciousness to spring forward to positive thoughts and allow the healing energy of the universe to flow once again through your body and mind.

Affirmations

It is always remarkable to me how powerful your words can be in shaping your actions and your life. I am a firm believer that your body will follow what you say you are. So if you are a person who suffers from chronic pain, you might not realize that what you say could be perpetuating your suffering as much as your thoughts. As you go through your day, try to see yourself from the outside and actually listen to the words you use to describe yourself and your various situations in your life, from your job, to your relationships, to your perception of your own existence. You might find that you are actually saying out loud that you won't get better, you are destined to be in pain, or that it is your fate to be afflicted.

By using affirmations to change your spoken words about your perceived life situations, you can create powerful forces of change that your body will eventually follow. I like to have my patients write down their affirmations and say them in the mirror while looking themselves in the eye. Repeat them every morning before brushing your teeth and every evening before going to bed, and you will find your words will change your life. Say them with conviction and the changes you desire will come more quickly. I always recommend my patients read Louise Hay's great book, *You Can Heal Your Life*, to get a more in-depth analysis of the power of affirmations. I have included here some great affirmations for women with pelvic pain, but it is also great if you write some of your own as well. Remember to write your affirmations in the present tense with words like "I am," or "I have", so your mind can tell your body that these are states of life that you already are in, not some distant place where you hope to be in the future.

Table 15.2: Affirmations for Pelvic Pain

AFFIRMATION
1. I am healed.
2. I am having great and pain-free sex with my partner.
3. I have supple, soft and pain-free pelvic floor muscles.
4. I am surrounded by love.
5. I am in a loving and satisfying relationship.
6. I have a beautiful baby who came to me as a result of a beautiful birth.

Keep It Simple: Stop Taking on Too Much

Are you taking on too much work or find yourself overscheduled? Are you not sure how to say *no* to other people's demands on your time? If the answer is *yes*, than you can put yourself in a state of chronic stress and you habitually will tend to take on more than you can handle. Do you find you are constantly putting yourself last on your own list? If this is the case you might be subconsciously sabotaging your healing and causing yourself undue stress, tension and pressure.

If you are constantly telling yourself you just don't have time to do your Renew Program for Women™ healing techniques, then you have to break the cycle of taking on too much. If you have to, schedule time for yourself during the day and in the mornings and evenings. Even 15 minutes during the day to do a quick mediation, breathing, mantra, and workplace stretching program will work wonders for your body, mind, and soul. You will also find that once you begin to carve out time for yourself, it becomes easier to keep on doing it because your body and your mind will gravitate to the positive way it makes you feel.

Tips for Keeping It Simple and Not Taking on Too Much

1. Say no to family and friends if it puts you under stress.

2. Make sure that your work schedule does not interfere with your healing work.

3. Space out your social calendar so that you have ME time.

4. Do something that brings you joy and happiness everyday, even if it is as simple as looking at flowers for 5 minutes.

5. Surround yourself with positive energy and avoid being around negative people.

Join a Self-Help Group

I find that the women that do the best in my practice have someone to talk to about their emotional pain. Many of my patients tell me they feel better and less stressed after being surrounded by women who have the same problems as they do. They also tell me that having a sex therapist or psychoanalyst to talk to can be healing, helpful and keeps them positive.

TIPS:

1. Join a self-help group and keep with it for several months.

2. Get a life-coach.

3. See a psychotherapist or a sex therapist for your emotional pain.

4. If there are no groups near you, then start one yourself or join an Internet blog.

5. Ask your physical therapist if she could help you arrange a self-help group with other patients.

Gratitude Training - Rock and Walk

When I first saw *The Secret* by Rhonda Byrnes I was captured by the part in the DVD when they mentioned having an "Attitude of Gratitude." Another great source for gratitude training is Deepak Chopra, who talks about gratitude and how it needs to be the foundation of your overall outlook. I constantly find that my patients come to me and are so focused on their pain and how it pervades their whole life that it is the only thing on their minds. I always tell them, although they often look at me like I am crazy at first, that they need to think about all of the things they are grateful for instead. I tell them that in order to get on the road to healing, they have to first focus on things that are positive in their lives instead of focusing only on the pain and what they don't have.

Gratitude Rocks

When my patients come to me on their first visit I give them a gratitude rock. This rock is to remind them of the beauty, love and joy that they currently have in their lives.

WHAT TO DO:

1. Find a rock small enough that you can carry with you everyday. I carry mine in my pocket or purse. I collect rocks from the ocean or streams because they are smooth and have all of the rough and symbolically "painful edges" smoothed off by the power of water. I let my patients pick a rock that captures their eye.

2. When you are having a hard day and a pain flare-up, touch your rock and repeat to yourself: "I am grateful today for _____." Think about your statement and feel it. Feel the joy, happiness and elation around your statement. Send these feelings to all your cells, all body parts and muscles.

3. Put the rock next to your bed, and when you wake up, roll up and sit on the edge of your bed. Take your rock in your hand and think about something you are grateful for. Set the tone for your day as one of gratitude, one in which your pain and negativity, if it comes, will only be a fleeting part of your day.

4. Remember that the universe will not give more than you can bear, so stay grateful for things as simple as having enough air to breathe, and you will have a powerful transformational effect on your existence.

Gratitude Walks

As part of your cardiovascular training, incorporate gratitude into your walking program. Be conscious of how your thoughts are taking up space in your mind while you are walking, and make sure to take notice of the beauty around you. If you are walking in the park, take notice of birds, flowers, kids playing, the sunlight shining through the trees, or any other visuals or sounds that should make you feel grateful. Instead of thinking about how much you hate your boss or how much pain you are in, think about how grateful you are to be working at all, and how grateful you are to be on the road to healing, even if you are currently only making the smallest of steps forward in your program. The momentum will build and you will be amazed at the results.

The Present Moment - Staying in the Power of Now

Misery, stress and unhappiness are usually caused by thinking about events that are in the future or in the past. I find that when my patients stay present "in the now" they have less stress and anxiety. A personal favorite is Eckhart Tolle, a great author and lecturer who has written many books including a wonderful book called *The Power of Now*. I recommend this book to my patients, and they tell me they now understand how the constant flurry of activity that occurs in their minds affects their health and overall outlook. It is not difficult to be in the present but you must make an effort to be in the now.

Tolle talks at length about how the mind creates "the story of me," and how your ego tries to interpret events and actions in your life within this context. So if your mind has created a story of me that is one of perpetual pain, then your mind and ego will seek out events and people and interpretations of what has happened to you to keep going with this story. Once you let go of the past and the future, which are only creations of the mind, you can embrace the present moment, which you will find is actually quite manageable and one in which you can make conscious decisions to move forward down the path to your ultimate healing.

TIPS:

1. When thinking about future events or past events bring your mind to the present moment and focus your energy on your current breath. You can acknowledge your thoughts and thank your brain for trying to interpret every perception in the context of "the story of me," but let your mind know that you are going to focus on the present moment right now and enjoy it without interpretation.

2. Get a copy of Eckhart Tolle's book, *The Power of Now*, and read it at least 2 times.

Creative Visualizations

As discussed earlier, you are what you think and say you are, so be careful because the universe will lovingly give you what you think and declare you are. So why not start by thinking and visualizing yourself well, free from excess mental chatter, happy, and pain-free. Creative visualization is a great tool to use to reduce stress related to your painful condition. It's quite easy to do and can consist of almost any visualization. Below are 2 examples I have found that work great for my patients.

The Mirrored Hallway

Several times a day, whenever you are able, take a moment for a mental break and try the mirrored hallway visualization exercise. Repeat the exercise at least once per day for 2 to 4 weeks and track your progress. You should begin to see just how powerful your mind can be in keeping you in a state of pain if you let it, even subconsciously keeping you from declaring that you are better each day.

WHAT TO DO:

1. This exercise can be done sitting or lying down. I like to do this on the subway on my way home.

2. Close your eyes and focus on your breathing for 5 breaths. Focus on slowing down your breathing. Release the thoughts of the day up until that point, inhale through the nose and exhale through the mouth. Don't think about the future or the past.

3. Imagine the lights are being turned on and you find yourself in a short 6 to 8 foot hallway with a door on one end. You are just entering the hallway so the door is at the other end of the hallway.

4. You then notice that there are floor to ceiling mirrors on both sides of the hallway. On the left, see yourself or your situation, allowing your reflection

to be your state of pain, your misery, your negative outlook, anything in life which you wish to overcome.

5. Then look to the right and allow your reflection to be the exact opposite from the left. See yourself in a pain-free state, happy, filled with positive thoughts, having overcome that which your mind tells you you cannot overcome. Focus and remember how good you will feel since you have overcome your pain.

6. Then turn back to the left mirror, notice that there is a large wooden staff in the corner of the hallway. Take the staff and smash the mirror on the left in one forceful blow, bringing your mind into that moment, telling your mind that you will not tolerate these reflections to exist any longer.

7. Focus back on the right, and then walk through the hall seeing your reflection, open the door and continue on your journey as a pain-free person.

Mental Suds Visualization

I like to use this visualization as a gauge to help me get a sense of how many thoughts are actually "on my mind." At first you will find how amazingly filled your mind is even when you think you are in the moment. I often use this visualization as I prepare to do a meditation and mantra to calm down my mind.

WHAT TO DO:

1. Sit comfortably, with your eyes closed, with your focus slightly upward towards your third eye. Your third eye is the area above your nose and in between your eyebrows.

2. Allow the thoughts in your head to flow freely into this area of focus. Don't worry if the thoughts are good or bad, simply take notice of them as they cross your focus.

3. As each thought passes into your gaze, place it into a bubble and allow it to float in your perception. Don't let it float away, but keep it within your gaze.

4. Repeat this for each thought that is currently "on your mind." You may find in a short while that all of the bubbles you have created have made what I call "mental suds," where the bubbles are so close together that they look like suds in a bubble bath. If this is the case, don't worry; you have just created a mental picture of what is whizzing through your mind at the present moment.

5. Make an effort to pop bubbles in your field of view, releasing the thoughts contained in each bubble which are not important to your present moment.

6. Try to pop all the bubbles that relate to your past or to things you have to do or that relate to relationships and how you need to talk to this person or that person, or how you are always going to be in pain, etc. Leave just a couple of bubbles in your field of view, maybe one bubble filled with a thought about your breath and how it can heal you, and maybe another bubble filled with a thought about something you are grateful for, and maybe one bubble with a thought about how great it is to be pain-free.

Part 5
New Approaches for Tough Conditions: Pudendal Neuralgia, Coccygodynia, Core, and Bladder

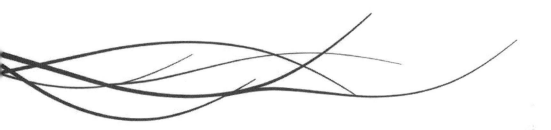

"Courage doesn't always roar. Sometimes courage is the little voice at the end of the day that says I'll try again tomorrow."
— Mary Anne Radmacher

Chapter Sixteen

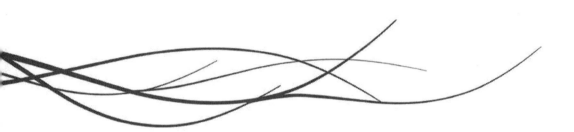

*"The difference between the possible
and the impossible lies in a man's determination."*
- Tommy Lasorda

Chapter 16

PUDENDAL NEURALGIA

Conditions involving the pudendal nerve are extremely complicated and extremely difficult to treat and manage. They are associated with impaired quality of life and high healthcare costs. For women with pudendal nerve conditions the price is high: many suffer from anxiety, depression and serious and debilitating pain. These individuals need help and clarity and a team of trained medical professionals in their corner. Many have been from doctor to doctor in search of answers; many have put themselves through medications, injections, MRI, CAT scans, nerve testing, etc. Although there is much confusion about pudendal nerve conditions, I am happy to report that there is movement now to distinguish between conditions that involve the pudendal nerve (PN). There are three conditions involving the pudendal nerve: 1) pudendal nerve neuralgia (PNN), a shooting, stabbing and knife-like pain in the distribution of the pudendal nerve; 2) pudendal nerve entrapment (PNE), an entrapment or compression of the pudendal nerve via muscles, fascia and ligaments; and 3) pudendal nerve canal syndrome (PNC), an issue of the nerve as it travels within Alcock's canal and becomes irritated, compressed or entrapped.

The pudendal nerve has a very unique anatomy and journey within the pelvic rim. Its journey makes it vulnerable to becoming entrapped, compressed or irritated by fascia, muscles, scar tissue, ligaments and surgeries of the pelvis. The tools in this chapter target PNN; one of the leading causes of PNN is myofascial dysfunction and the techniques described here work beautifully on these types of restrictions. Physical therapists successfully treat the pain, spasms, tight muscles, trigger points, connective tissue restrictions, scars and joint dysfunction that contribute to symptoms of PNN.

The hallmark sign for both PNE and PNN is pain that increases with sitting. Keep in mind, however, that not all pain that increases with sitting is attributable to a pudendal nerve that is entrapped or compressed. This hallmark sign led to the over-diagnosing of PNE; back in the 1980s every patient that came in with increased sitting pain was diagnosed with PNE. PNN and PNE were not as clearly delineated then as they are today. There was much confusion between the two and many patients were treated incorrectly, ineffectively or with surgeries that did not produce desired results. Today there are more knowledgeable medical professionals who can distinguish between the two and provide proper care and treatment. It's important to seek those caregivers who have firsthand experience in treating pudendal nerve conditions. Unfortunately, young doctors are sometimes baffled with these diagnoses. Better training regarding the pelvis and PFMs needs to occur in medical school so that women can find help more quickly instead of suffering for years with these conditions. Gynecologists and urologists in particular need to be well acquainted with this nerve, its path and clinical presentation. A woman's pudendal nerve can become injured during gynecological surgeries that include repairs for rectocele, cystocele and hysterectomies. Childbirth can also result in injuries of the pudendal nerve. OB/ GYNs should be on the lookout for clinical signs related to PNN so that young moms can get help more quickly and be referred to appropriate caregivers. Too often I treat PNN secondary to a perineal repair, perineal laceration or episiotomy. I know all too well that childbirth is unpredictable; my point is that women need the appropriate care and it needs to be given immediately. It is unfair to tell new moms they will heal from these complications of childbirth when every clinical sign points to conditions involving the pudendal nerve.

Additionally the pudendal nerve can be injured during bike riding, falls, ac- cidents, coccyx injuries, etc. Once the nerve becomes entrapped, injured or aggravated it can create horrific, deep and agonizing pain requiring the expertise of several trained medical professionals. It takes a village to help women with conditions relating to the pudendal nerve. Physical therapists in particular are an essential part of this medical team as we are experts in myofascial components of PNN including, but not limited to, sacroiliac joint corrections, PFM manipulations, connective tissue restrictions and trigger point releases. Women's health physical therapists who are trained to work with PNN can educate the patient on behavioral modifications and lifestyle changes, helping women in ways that other medical professionals cannot. PNN has many faces and can present in many ways that physical therapists are uniquely able to understand. Physical therapists are able to connect the dots and find the source of the PNN pain.

An injured pudendal nerve can cause pain in the labia, pain in the clitoris, pain in the perineal area, pain in the genital and perianal areas. The pudendal nerve serves numerous areas within the female pelvis, and pain anywhere in this area can probably be traced back to some sort of dysfunction of PN. Some of my patients with pudendal nerve conditions report feeling as if their pubic hair is being pulled or yanked out; others report anal burning and feeling as if there is something inside the vagina or rectum. Other women cannot tolerate wearing clothes against their privates and others state that their sit bones are on fire. Often sitting is impossible. To resolve conditions related to pudendal nerve issues you may need to work with a team that includes a physical therapist with pelvic floor specialty, a urogynecologist, a urologist, pain-management doctors, neurologists and surgeons. Partnership healthcare is extremely important and an absolute must when trying to resolve this condition. It can take up to one year of physical therapy treatments to achieve desired results. Women have to be proactive and do their self-care as described within this chapter. This information is not to be used in isolation but in conjunction with the rest of the care that you receive from your medical team including your trained physical therapist.

I've had tremendous success in treating PNN pain with physical therapy techniques. I have seen dramatic decreases in pain and tremendous improvement in everyday functioning. Treating PNN is an art form and I intend to give you a broad understanding so you can help and treat yourself. You must be able to connect all the dots because this nerve can express itself anywhere within the pelvic region and the more dots you connect the better and more effective your self-healing therapies will be. Palpation skills and knowing the external access to the pudendal nerve will be extremely helpful, so please review all the anatomy in this book. A whole mind/body approach is something that you, your physical therapist and other medical providers will have to adopt to succeed with pudendal nerve conditions. Please make sure to acquaint yourself with the mind/body chapter in this book and choose the exercises that help you to stay relaxed and positive.

The symptoms related to pudendal nerve conditions vary widely. According to Dr. Jacques Beco there are three clinical signs of pudendal *neuropathy*. (Dr. Beco uses the term *neuropathy* instead of PNE and PNN because it simply states that there is something wrong with the pudendal nerve but the cause is unknown. I personally like the term *pudendal neuropathy* but for clarification purposes I used PNN and PNE in this chapter.) He states the clinical signs of pudendal neuropathy include:

1. Perineal hypo- or hyperesthesia (pinprick);
2. Painful pudendal nerve during vaginal/rectal examination; and
3. Painful skin rolling test of the perineal skin.

There are other clinical signs that can be used such as an old-fashioned physical therapy Tinel's sign of pudendal nerve. To perform a Tinel test on the pudendal nerve, you must be palpated either rectally or vaginally and gently tap the nerve. It is best to leave this test to a professional so you don't risk hurting yourself. Positive Tinel test results include pain in the distribution of the nerve and this test indicates there's an issue with the nerve. While not indicative of PNE, the Tinel test does show that the nerve is involved. Of course you can also palpate the pudendal nerve to see if there's tenderness. I normally do this intra-vaginally at ischial spine.

There are other clinical criteria of which you should also be aware, such as Nantes criteria. Nantes criteria was established to diagnose PNN as it relates to PNE. There are no specific tests that can positively show that an individual has PNN or PNE, but Nantes criteria is a clinical tool that facilitates the diagnosis of PNN by PNE. Nantes criteria includes five clinical findings and they must all be present to point the finger toward PNN by PNE. While the only way to diagnose PNN by PNE conclusively is via surgery, many MDs use Nantes criteria. Nantes criteria include:

1. Pain in the distribution of the pudendal nerve;
2. Pain that is increased and predominantly found with sitting;
3. The pain does not keep the patient awake at night;
4. No objective sensory impairments are found; and
5. Administration of a pudendal block relieves pain.

In addition to the clinical signs, listen carefully to your symptoms as they will point you to tools in this book that can help you overcome this type of pelvic pain. You need to work directly on the PFMs to restore their function, tone and coordination. Success with PNN depends on intravaginal and intrarectal work on the PFMs. You must become an expert in treating yourself and in finding trigger points in the pelvic floor including the obturator internus muscle. External trigger points must be resolved and eliminated and the pelvic and sacroiliac joint must be aligned for optimal functioning.

Give special attention to pain in the sacroiliac joint and the pelvic rim bones. Any misalignment issues here will have a profound effect on the pudendal nerve. For sacroiliac dysfunction corrections I use muscle energy techniques (MET) as they help to maintain the body in good form and help reduce tension on the pudendal nerve itself. I will not be covering MET here because it is beyond the scope of this book, but please consider taking a class or reading a book on this topic. Also become familiar with the symptoms and causes relating to PNN. I have listed them in Table 16.2 and Table 16.3.

Additionally ask yourself about traumatic injuries or falls that may have happened to you in your life, including childhood injuries. The information you gather will help establish a treatment plan that includes many of the techniques already covered in this book. In the next sections I will share with you common complaints, common causes of pudendal nerve injury, anatomy and healing techniques I use on women suffering from PNN.

Anatomy and Journey of the Pudendal Nerve

Relevant Pudendal Nerve Information

The pudendal nerve has a long and winding path within the pelvic rim area. The pudendal nerve originates at ventral rami nerve roots of S2 through S4. The pudendal nerve travels within the pelvic region in three different places that include the gluteal region, pudendal canal (Alcock's canal) and perineum. Please note that the pudendal nerve also travels within the greater and lesser sciatic foramen. The greater and lesser sciatic foramen are formed by the sacrospinous and sacrotuberous ligament. These ligaments can sometimes pinch and/or compress this nerve. The path of this nerve makes it vulnerable not only to compression but also to injury. There are four areas where the nerve can be compressed, irritated and/or injured. They include:

1. Underneath the piriformis muscle,
2. Between the sacrospinous and scarotuberous ligaments,
3. Pudendal canal, and
4. Where the dorsal nerve of the clitoris emerges from underneath the inferior ramus of the pubic bone and turns cephalad (toward the head).

For clarity I want you to understand the sites where the nerve can be compressed. Please note that PNE cannot be diagnosed with your standard MRI. Many of my patients have gotten a PNE diagnosis after getting an MRI only to discover that it's really PNN pain they are experiencing. A diagnosis of PNE is a very serious matter and should not be taken lightly. It is important to set realistic goals and expectations. Women suffering from pudendal nerve conditions will undergo physical therapy and self-healing care anywhere from six months to one to two years. To normalize the body of those who suffer from pudendal nerve conditions takes time. You may need to consider injections, painkillers and muscle relaxers. I see these modalities as a temporary solution to get you to the next phase of healing. Some of my patients learn how to take care of themselves and develop their own treatment plans for flare-ups. Be sure to work with a specialist who is open to your needs and suggestions.

Diagram 16.1: Anatomy of the Pudendal Nerve

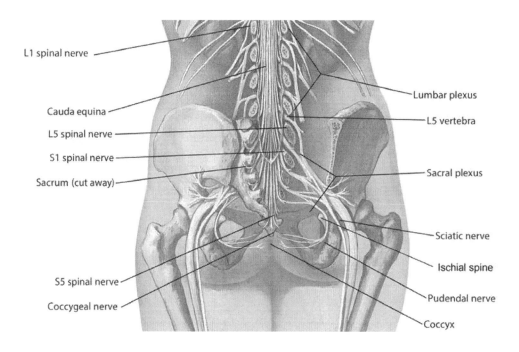

Diagram description: Notice the anatomy and how the pudendal nerve loops around the ischial spine. Source: Netter Images

Diagram 16.2: Anterior View of the Sacral Area

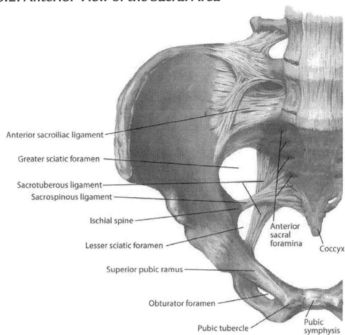

Anterior sacroiliac ligament

Greater sciatic foramen

Sacrotuberous ligament
Sacrospinous ligament

Ischial spine

Lesser sciatic foramen

Superior pubic ramus

Obturator foramen

Pubic tubercle

Anterior
sacral
foramina

Coccyx

Pubic
symphysis

Diagram Description: Notice the sacral tuberous and sacral spinous ligament. Source: Netter Images

The Pudendal Nerve Journey

1. The ventral rami of nerve roots S2 to S4 join to form the pudendal nerve trunk. The pudendal nerve is a mixed nerve with sensory, motor and autonomic fibers.

2. The pudendal nerve travels laterally and inferiorly on the anterior surface of the piriformis muscle. (This can explain why many patients who suffer from pudendal nerve neuropathy complain about deep gluteal pain and have numerous trigger points in the gluteal muscles.)

3. After leaving the piriformis muscle it is joined by the internal pudendal artery and vein. They travel downward together for a short course in the pelvis before exiting the pelvis via greater sciatic foramen.

4. The pudendal nerve then loops around the sacrospinous ligament and ischial spine. This is a common site where the pudendal nerve can become compressed, entrapped or irritated. It re-enters the perineum via the lesser sciatic foramen. Note that the nerve also travels between the sacrospinous ligament and sacrotuberous ligament. These two ligaments can clamp down and compress this nerve causing pain and symptoms of PNN.

5. The pudendal nerve then gives off one of its three branches, the inferior anal branch (rectal nerve). The branching of the pudendal nerve is variable and can occur at different sites. The rectal branch can come off:

    1. Beneath or through the sacrotuberous ligament;

    2. Through the sacrospinous ligament;

    3. It can travel within the pudendal canal;

    4. It can branch off after the pudendal nerve exits the pudendal canal; or

    5. It can branch off directly at the sacral plexus and reconnect with the pudendal nerve or run independently to the anus. As you can see, it is difficult to say with certainty where the branching of the rectal nerve will occur. The rectal nerve innervates the external anal sphincter, the distal anal canal, and the circumanal skin and may supply sensory branches to the lower part of the vagina.

6. The pudendal nerve then enters the pudendal canal within the ischioanal fossa traveling from its posterior (buttock) to anterior (pubis) position through a space formed by the connective tissue (fascia) that covers the pudendal artery/vein. This connective tissue or aponeurosis of the obturator internus was first described by Alcock and is termed Alcock's canal, (currently known as the pudendal canal). There is a posterior entrance to the canal and an anterior exit from the canal. This is important because the nerve can become entrapped, compressed or irritated in this canal.

7. The pudendal nerve within the pudendal canal gives off another two additional terminal branches, the perineal branch and the dorsal nerve to the

clitoris. My research shows this branching occurs within the canal; there are likely anomalies here as well.

8. The second branch, the perineal branch of the pudendal nerve, runs inferiorly in Alcock's canal, dividing into the posterior labial (sensory) branch and muscular (motor) branch. The posterior labial branch travels in the lateral part of the urogenital triangle and supplies the skin of the labia majora and the skin of the lower vagina. The motor branch innervates the superficial transverse perineal muscle, ischiocavernosus, bulbospongiosus, external anal sphincter, and deep transverse perineal.

Diagram 16.3: Innervation of the External Female Genitalia: The Pudendal Nerve

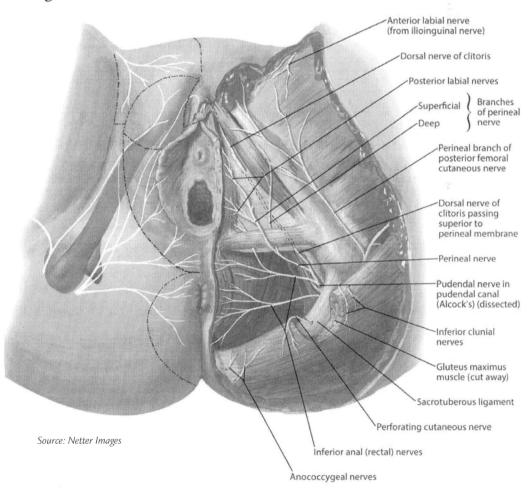

Anterior labial nerve (from ilioinguinal nerve)

Dorsal nerve of clitoris

Posterior labial nerves

Superficial } Branches of perineal nerve
Deep

Perineal branch of posterior femoral cutaneous nerve

Dorsal nerve of clitoris passing superior to perineal membrane

Perineal nerve

Pudendal nerve in pudendal canal (Alcock's) (dissected)

Inferior clunial nerves

Gluteus maximus muscle (cut away)

Sacrotuberous ligament

Perforating cutaneous nerve

Inferior anal (rectal) nerves

Anococcygeal nerves

Source: Netter Images

9. The third branch, the dorsal clitoral nerve, appears from underneath the inferior ramus of the pubic bone and penetrates into the urogenital membrane. It then turns sharply cephalad, traveling between the ischiocavernosus muscle and inferior margin of the inferior pubic ramus. This is another area where the nerve can become entrapped and or irritated. The nerve then makes a very sharp anterior turn entering the clitoris. It is here where the nerve begins dividing into its smaller terminal branches.

Table 16.1: Branches of Pudendal Nerve and Areas of Innervation

PUDENDAL NERVE BRANCHES	AREAS OF INNERVATION
Dorsal Nerve of the Clitoris	**Clitoris** • Ischiocavernosus • Bulbospongiosus • (Possible cross innervations because of close proximity. The author invites you to research further.)
Perineal Branch	**Sensory Branch** • Lower inferior third of the vagina and urethra • Skin of labia majora **Motor Branch** • Superficial transverse perineal muscle • Ischiocavernosus • Bulbospongiosus • External anal sphincter (anterior portion) • Urethral sphincter
Inferior Rectal Branch	• Distal anal canal • Circumanal skin • Sensory branches to the lower vagina • External anal sphincter muscle (posterior portion)

Table 16.2: Symptoms Associated with Pudendal Nerve Conditions

SYMPTOMS ASSOCIATED WITH PUDENDAL NERVE CONDITIONS
Abnormal temperature sensations
Anal burning, itching or pain
A feeling like the pubic hairs are being pulled or yanked
Burning with urination
Clitoral hypersensitivity
Clitoral pain with or without contact
Constipation
Deep ache in the vagina
Dyspareunia
Fecal incontinence
Feeling tensed muscles and/or spasms in the vagina
Feeling of a lump or foreign body inside the vagina
Enlarged vulvar veins
Hyperarousal syndrome—arousal without sexual contact or thoughts (PGAD)
Numbness or loss of sensation in the perianal and genital areas
Pain in the vulva or clitoris with contact or oral sex
Pain with sitting that gets worse as the day progresses
Pain with sitting that is reduced when sitting on the toilet
Pain with bowel movements
Pain that increases with bending forward or lifting heavy objects or children
Pain in the perineum (area between the anus and vagina)
Pain with wearing underwear or pants
Pain with sexual intercourse
Pain in the lower back, groin, buttocks
Pain in posterior thigh, calf and/or ankle
Pelvic floor muscle spasms

Table CONTINUES on next page

Table 16.2: Symptoms Associated with Pudendal Nerve Conditions

CONTINUED from previous page

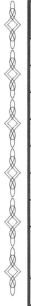

SYMPTOMS ASSOCIATED WITH PUDENDAL NERVE CONDITIONS
Persistent Genital Arousal Disorder (PGAD)
Proctalgia fugax
Post-orgasm pain either immediately or within hours or days
Spinal cord or nerve root compression
Sexual dysfunction such as diminished orgasms or difficulty achieving orgasms
Sit-bone pain and/or burning sensation
Spontaneous orgasms without sexual contact
Stabbing, shooting or burning pain in the pelvis, anus, labia, and in any other area that the pudendal nerve innervates
Stress incontinence
Vestibule pain, burning, itching
Urge incontinence
Urinary frequency/urgency/hesitancy

Table 16.3: Possible Causes of Pudendal Nerve-Related Conditions

POSSIBLE CAUSES OF PUDENDAL NERVE-RELATED CONDITIONS
Childbirth trauma
Vaginal and pelvic surgeries or prolapse repair surgeries
Biking
Prolonged sitting or prolonged sitting in poor posture
Connective tissue and fascial restrictions
Perineal descent and anal prolapse increase stretch on pudendal nerve
Polyneuropathy from diabetes
Traumatic (and sometimes not so traumatic) injuries
Falls on the coccyx
Car accidents where the spine has a direct hit
Severe pelvic floor muscle spasms
Prolonged straining with constipation
Heavy weightlifting and squatting
Hysterectomy
Previous infections
Repetitive minor traumas or injuries
Sacroiliac dysfunction
Pelvic rim misalignment issues can influence the path of the pudendal nerve
Pelvic floor muscle spasms
Pelvic floor tension myalgia
Post-partum hematoma with or without subsequent scar tissue
Traction of the legs during orthopedic surgeries
Heavy manipulations by osteopaths, chiropractors and other practitioners
Fibrosis of the ischioanal fossa
Iatrogenic, caused by medical examination or treatment, such as intravaginal injections

Table 16.4: Recommended Activity Modification and Lifestyle Changes: What to Avoid

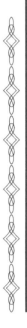

RECOMMENDED ACTIVITY MODIFICATION AND LIFESTYLE CHANGES: WHAT TO AVOID
Initially avoid excessively over-stretching the piriformis muscle.
Avoid exercises that bring on your pain.
Avoid constipation or urinary problems.
Avoid prolonged sitting; pay attention to your sitting tolerance and if necessary get a standing desk.
Avoid hamstring stretching especially with the knees straight.
Avoid dead lifts.
Avoid improper ergonomics for computer and work stations.
Avoid squatting and loading the shoulders with weight while squatting at the gym.
Avoid certain yoga poses that put excessive strain on nerves such as down dog, forward bends, single leg stretches, and hamstring stretches.
Avoid traditional sit-ups.
Avoid traditional Kegels.
Avoid inflammatory foods and drinks.
Avoid stress.
Avoid catastrophization of thoughts and pain.

Table 16.5: Recommended Activities and Lifestyle Changes

RECOMMENDED ACTIVITIES AND LIFESTYLE CHANGES
Use a cushion when sitting. Avoid sitting on yoga blocks and/or hard surfaces. Find a cushion that disperses the weight off the sit bones.
Set up your computer stations ergonomically. Never work with an improper computer set-up.
Incorporate reverse Kegels into your daily routine.
Use mind/body and breathing techniques to keep calm and relaxed. Meditation on a daily basis will do wonders for you.
Listen to your body and know what self-care tools get you out of pain. Don't override your pain signals.
Take daily warm baths if possible.
Keep your thoughts positive and focus on the good things in your life.
Question thoughts that are catastrophic and negative and turn them into positive thoughts. This is very difficult and takes time but questioning your thoughts for their validity will open up new possibilities for you.
Walking is great. Try to walk up to 30 minutes per day or as tolerated by your pain.
Swimming is highly recommended.
Try acupuncture therapy.
Focus on the things you can do instead of what you can no longer do and do those things with love and gusto. Find new hobbies that fulfill you as a person.
Remember to have hope and to always believe that you will get better.
Join a self-help group and/or seek professional care from a trained therapist.
Do sound healing therapy to get the stress and tension out of the body. This new modality is working wonders with many of my patients.
Energy healing and Reiki go a long way. These modalities are giving my patients favorable outcomes.

Healing Techniques and Self-Care Tools for Women Suffering from Pudendal Nerve Neuralgia

Listed below you will find some of the healing techniques I use with my patients. Remember to explore this book and try all the techniques to determine which ones will work for you. The rolling of the sacrum, sit bones, ischioanal fossa and the area between the sit bone and coccyx are critical in PNN. These areas are very close to each other often making it hard to distinguish these areas. You must know your landmarks and think about what you are doing here. Connective tissue rolling helps to improve circulation and provide oxygen to areas affected by PNN. It also helps reduce adverse tension on the pudendal nerve itself. Rolling also helps to restore connective tissue and muscle balance integrity. The rolling is best done without oil, but if this is too painful, use oil until you can tolerate rolling these areas without oil.

Ischioanal Fossa Anatomy

Ischioanal fossa is a wedge-shaped space on either side of the anal canal. The fossa's base is toward the perineum and it's situated between the sit bones and is bordered laterally by the obturator internus muscle and medially by the external anal sphincter and levator ani. This fossa houses important structures such as the pudendal canal, which contains the pudendal nerve, pudendal artery and pudendal vein. Ischioanal fossa also contains fat that expands to maintain continence and expands the anal canal when it has feces in it. When there's a dysfunction within this fossa it can lead to deep pelvic pain and pain that comes on with pressure such as sitting. Many times women will complain of burning in the sit bones, numbness, pubic hair pulling, burning in the vestibule, incontinence and pain that is relentless and unprovoked or provoked with sitting.

Table 16.6: Ischioanal Fossa Anatomy

AREA	BORDERS
Anterior	- Urogenital triangle and its fascia - Deep transverse perineal muscle
Lateral	- Sit bones - Obturator muscle - Obturator fascia and pudendal canal
Superior	- Levator Ani muscles
Inferior	- Skin - Superficial fascia
Medial	- Levator Ani muscles - External anal sphincter muscle - Anal fascia
Posterior	- Sacrotuberous ligament - Gluteus maximus

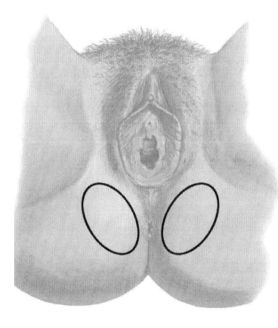

Source: Netter Images

Ischioanal Rolling

The circles indicate where the ischioanal rolling should be performed.

WHAT TO DO:

1. The ischioanal fossa has several borders and the treatment of this area with rolling and massaging cannot be overstated or overlooked.

2. Locate the ischioanal fossa between the sit bone and the anal rim; palpate the soft tissue cavity.

3. Place your fingerstips in the lower part of the fossa and the thumbs on the upper part. The idea is to roll the skin of the fossa toward the thumbs. Roll this area up to five minutes. Focus on the most painful side first.

4. You can do this exercise by gripping the fossa underneath the butt check and rolling it upward toward the sit bone.

Sit-Bone Connective Tissue Rolling

You might have a hard time performing this technique on yourself if you are lying down. I find that the best way to do this on myself is in a standing position.

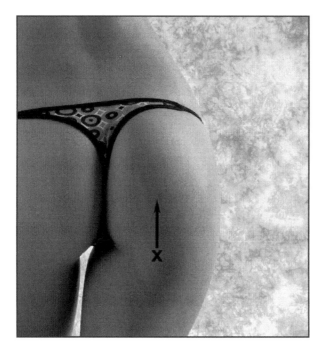

WHAT TO DO:

1. Stand with your feet hip-width apart and knees in a bent position. Lean against the wall with the left hand for support.

2. Place the fingertips of your right hand under the sit-bone area and your thumb on the lower part of your gluteal muscles.

3. Gently roll the connective tissue of the sit bone area upward toward the gluteal muscles.

Ligament Rolling (Between Sit Bone and Coccyx Bone)

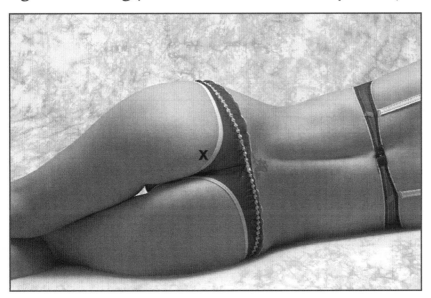

You might have a hard time performing this technique on yourself if you are lying down. I find that the best way to do this on myself is in a standing position or in a side-lying position.

GETTING STARTED:

Find the bony landmarks of the coccyx and the sit bone. This is a very small area.

WHAT TO DO:

1. Cup your fingertips and place them at your coccyx. Roll this area toward your sit bones.

2. Roll for up to five minutes or as tolerated.

Sacral Rolling

I love this technique because it brings profound pain relief while restoring neurological, connective tissue and bony functions. This is the area from where the pudendal nerve arises and we want to keep it free of restrictions. It is also included earlier in the book but is repeated because it provides great relief for PNN.

GETTING STARTED:

The sacrum houses many of the nerve roots that innervate the abdominal organs, PFMs and hip muscles. It is critical to keep the tissues in this area free and supple. Sacral rolling is a great tool for this.

WHAT TO DO:

1. Cup the skin in your sacral area and roll it in the same manner that you would roll your abdominals. See the photo for hand placement.

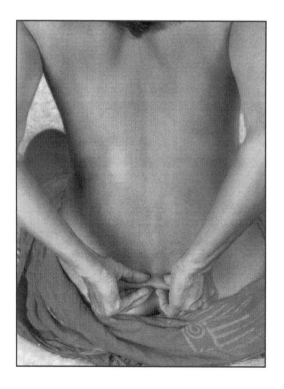

2. Roll the sacrum upward for two to five minutes on a daily basis. In the beginning, sacral rolling might be painful, but over time it will become less painful.

3. The goal is to be pain-free when doing the sacral rolling.

Anal Rim Massage

I included this technique here again as well as it can be very effective for PNN, which can often result in rectal pain and constipation. To reduce pain and reduce tension on the anal PFMs I massage the anal rim area. PNN sometimes results in anal itching and burning and this simple technique can help reduce these symptoms.

WHAT TO DO:

1. Spread the buttocks to reveal the anus.

2. Slowly and gently massage the rim using circular motions in a clockwise direction only.

3. You can use some type of organic oil for this massage.

4. You can massage the anal rim for three to five minutes or as tolerated. Get as close to the anus as possible. If you have external hemorrhoids this technique might not be for you. Proceed with caution or don't do it at all. Rubbing external hemorrhoids might cause them to bleed or get worse.

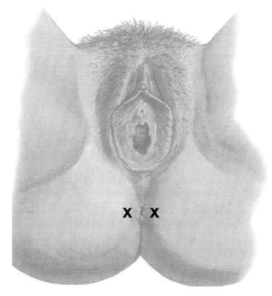

Base Image Source: Netter Images

Piriformis Massage and Trigger Point Release

The piriformis muscle lies centrally in the gluteal region and the pudendal nerve travels anteriorly to this muscle. It is very important to keep this muscle tension free and without trigger points.

WHAT TO DO:

1. Explore the piriformis muscle and massage this muscle from the sacrum to the hip bone.

2. While you are massaging the piriformis muscle, be on the lookout for trigger points. Press into any trigger point and hold from 30 to 90 seconds or until the pain diminishes by 50 percent. For specifics on trigger point work see Chapter 10.

3. You can also foam roll this muscle (Chapter 8) and use the tennis ball technique (Chapter 14).

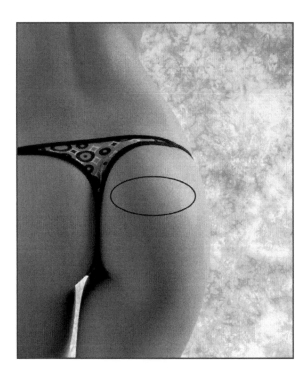

Intravaginal Massage and Trigger Point Release of the Obturator Internus Muscle

The obturator internus muscle is a hip external rotator that you can access via the vagina or rectum. The fascia of the obturator internus muscle creates the pudendal canal. This muscle must be targeted internally with intravaginal techniques to restore pudendal nerve function, release muscular tension, spasms and trigger points within it. The techniques highlighted include PFM half-moon strumming, myofascial release and trigger point release; all will help release the obturator internus and restore its function.

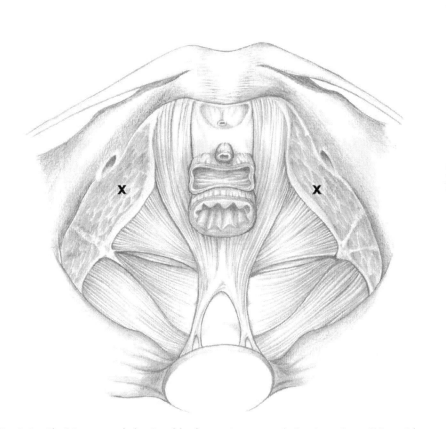

Description: The "x" represents the location of the obturator internus muscle. Base Image Source: Winston Johnson.

GETTING STARTED:

1. To find the obturator internus muscle insert your finger up to the third knuckle and bend the tip of the finger in a "come hither" position toward the nine or three o'clock positions depending on the side of the body you are working. For this deep muscle I find that using a dilator or Crystal Wand works well. If you are not keen on using a dilator or Crystal Wand, lie on your side and use your thumb. I find this to be a better alternative position for working on the obturator internus muscle.

2. Confirm that you are on the obturator internus muscle and not on one of the PFMs. Do this by moving your thigh outward and resisting this outward rotation with your hand. The obturator internus will pop into your hand.

3. Work to resolve any trigger points in this muscle and massage to restore its muscle fiber length by performing the half-moon strumming massage.

4. You can also use cross friction on this muscle. My advice is to try all three methods in combination.

Restore PFM Health by Reducing Tension, Trigger Points and Spasms

Please read Chapter 9 and understand how to perform all the techniques listed in that chapter. Women with PNN suffer from pelvic floor muscle dysfunction and these muscles must be restored back to their vitality, strength, coordination and health. Work on all the layers of the PFMs as part of your strategy for PNN relief. Many times, symptoms of PNN improve or lessen by normalizing PFM function.

ADDITIONAL CLINICAL CONSIDERATIONS

There are many techniques that are beyond the scope of this book. I encourage you to work with a women's health physical therapist to ensure your therapy is well-rounded and targeted. Additional clinical considerations for physical therapists working with women suffering from PNN include the following:

- Align the sacroiliac joint, ilium, pubic bones, and coccyx.
- Stabilize sacroiliac joint, with exercise or belting.
- Normalize tension and spasms in all PFMs and improve PFM coordination.
- Normalize bowel and bladder function and if necessary put your patients on a bladder retraining program.
- Advise your patients about lifestyle changes and behavior modifications.
- Investigate and track their pain, changes in pain or pain patterns.
- Advise them as to ergonomics for work and home.
- Pudendal nerve glides as needed. Make sure to take a class or learn from a mentor before attempting to glide the pudendal nerve.
- Correct sitting posture and posture in general.
- Focus on reverse Kegels.
- Evaluate and mobilize the hips.
- Correct pelvic rim muscle imbalances.
- Resolve connective tissue and fascial restrictions.
- Appropriate medical workup including imaging.

Now that we have covered pudendal nerve conditions and self-care strategies, I want to touch on another major cause of pelvic pain that causes much confusion: tailbone pain or coccydynia. Many of the women we treat at our healing center suffer from tailbone pain. They usually come seeking pain relief and want to learn how they can avoid more pain and—most importantly—how they can help themselves. This next chapter covers coccydynia and provides many self-help tips and strategies. Read this chapter and evaluate the coccyx bone because a dysfunction here often leads to pain and/or dysfunction of the PFMs.

Chapter Seventeen

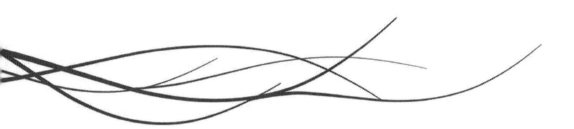

"Sometimes life hits you in the head with a brick. Don't lose faith."

- Steve Jobs

Chapter 17

COCCYDYNIA: HOW TO RELIEVE YOUR COCCYX PAIN ON YOUR OWN

Although the coccyx (tailbone) is a small bone, it is mighty and major repercussions result when it is injured, broken or misaligned. Additional causes of coccyx pain, also known as coccydynia, are spasms of the pelvic floor muscles, referred pain from the lumbar spine and/or sacroiliac joint. Patients have also reported an onset of this pain after prolonged sitting on a hard surface and/or prolonged biking. Poor sitting posture is another culprit in coccyx pain. Injuries to the coccyx bone have profound implications on functioning of the PFMs, gluteal nerves, muscles, fascia and ligaments.

At my center in New York City we see injuries to the tailbone all the time. These coccyx injuries can make sitting a living hell with pain so excruciating that I have seen it make both men and women cry. Many times we see a broken coccyx that resulted from either childbirth or delivery. The women that we treat at our center with pelvic pain sometimes also suffer from coccyx pain. We make it our business to evaluate the coccyx of everyone that comes through our doors because of the coccyx's deep influence on the PFMs. Coccydynia is poorly understood and many clinicians are baffled about how to treat it. In this chapter I will cover simple tools and exercises that can bring you profound pain relief.

The most important thing is to get an X-ray to rule out a broken coccyx. If your coccyx is broken certain precautions need to be taken to prevent making matters worse. A broken coccyx needs to heal and an MD should do a follow-up X-ray to determine healing and what manipulations can be performed on you by a trained physical therapist. If the coccyx is strained or misaligned, there are self-care techniques that you can do to improve your condition. Of course, there are always injections and surgeries, but I rarely find them necessary if the coccyx is handled and treated properly.

Relevant Coccyx Anatomy

The coccyx is a small bone at the end of the spine that resembles a tail. It is composed of three to five individual coccygeal vertebrae. Depending on the person's make-up, the coccygeal bones can be fused to make a single bone or sometimes the first coccygeal vertebra is separated from the other fused coccygeal bones. The coccyx has an unusual shape with the anterior coccyx bone being concave and the posterior coccyx being convex. The top of the coccyx articulates with the sacrum via the sacrococcygeal junction. This junction and the junctions between the coccygeal vertebrae have fibrocartilaginous discs that are similar to discs present in between spinal vertebrae. Anterior to the coccyx at the sacrococcygeal junction lies an unpaired sympathetic ganglion called ganglion impar (ganglion of Walther). This ganglion can be either very sensitive or overly active contributing to coccyx pain. The coccyx serves as a shock absorber and as a weight-bearing structure along with the sit bones. The coccyx bears more weight when a person sits and is leaning back or when the patient sits in a poor posture with a slumped back. The coccyx bone also serves as an important site for the attachments of muscles, ligaments and tendons. Many of the PFM muscles also insert into the coccyx bone. Surgeons and patients should remember these attachments when they consider surgical removal of the coccyx. See Table 17.2 and familiarize yourself with the structures that attach to the coccyx.

The coccyx has the ability to move but excessive movement can create instability and can lead to pain. Hypo-mobility—too little movement— or misalignment, such as too much flexion or extension, can also cause pain. The coccyx can flex (move anteriorly toward the front of the body) and the coccyx can extend (move posteriorly toward the back of the body). With the patients that I treat I commonly find a flexed coccyx that is stuck anteriorly. A coccyx that is deviated left or right can also cause pain. In this case women usually lean to the opposite side of the coccyx deviation to reduce pain.

Diagram 17.1: Coccyx Posterior View

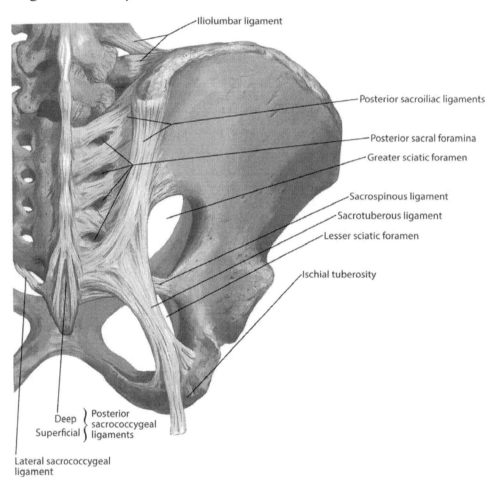

Iliolumbar ligament

Posterior sacroiliac ligaments

Posterior sacral foramina

Greater sciatic foramen

Sacrospinous ligament

Sacrotuberous ligament

Lesser sciatic foramen

Ischial tuberosity

Deep ⎫ Posterior
Superficial ⎬ sacrococcygeal
⎭ ligaments

Lateral sacrococcygeal
ligament

Description: Notice the complex web of ligaments in and around the coccyx. Some of the techniques in this book require that you work directly on these ligaments to eliminate coccyx pain. Source: Netter Images.

Table 17.1: Possible Causes of Coccyx Injuries

POSSIBLE CAUSES OF COCCYX INJURIES
Falling on the buttocks or falling backward onto the buttocks or sit bones
Childbirth in general as the baby can put pressure on the coccyx bone as it descends down the birth canal
Childbirth position such as the lithotomy position that encourages the coccyx to be overly flexed and for the baby to push up against it
Fracture to the coccyx bone after a traumatic fall
Gluteus maximus spasms
Inflammation
Pelvic floor muscle spasms
Referred pain from lumbar spine or sacroiliac joint
Traumatic injury
Tumor

Table 17.2: Bone Attachments of the Coccyx

COCCYX BONE ATTACHMENTS: MUSCLES, LIGAMENTS AND TENDONS
Gluteus maximus attaches to the posterior coccyx bone
Sacrospinous ligament fibers attach to the coccyx and connect the sacrum to the coccyx
Sacrotuberous ligament fibers attach to the coccyx and connect the sacrum to the coccyx
Ischiococcygeus (part of the PFMs)
Iliococcygeus (part of the PFMs)
Pubococcygeus (part of the PFMs)
Anococcygeal raphe: supports the position of the anus
Anterior and posterior sacrococcygeal ligaments attach the sacrum to the coccyx
External anal sphincter
Ganglion impar (unpaired sympathetic ganglion anterior to the sacrococcygeal junction)
Sacrococcygeal ligaments attached to the transverse process of the coccyx

Table 17.3: Symptoms of Coccydynia

SYMPTOMS OF COCCYDYNIA
Pain with sitting
Pain with going from a seated position to a standing position
Pain above the anus
Pain that improves with spinal extension such as leaning forward and sitting upright
Pain at the coccyx bone
Leaning to the side when sitting to take weight off a painful and/or deviated coccyx

Table 17.4: Conservative Strategies for the Pain Relief of Coccydynia

CONSERVATIVE STRATEGIES FOR THE PAIN RELIEF OF COCCYDYNIA
Use a donut or cushion when sitting. This takes weight off the coccyx and distributes it. A wedge cushion can also be used.
Sit upright in good posture and lean slightly forward to put the weight on the sit bones and not on the coccyx.
Lean to one side so your body weight is mostly on one sit bone.
Minimize your sitting and avoid activities that increase your coccyx pain.
Perform reverse Kegel exercises to get the coccyx to move posteriorly and to release tension and spasms in the PFMs.
Ice the coccyx and apply heat to the gluteal muscles.
Manual intrarectal or intravaginal mobilization by a trained physical therapist.
Releasing tightness and trigger points in the PFMs and associated muscles.
Lumbar spine exercises that help encourage coccyx movement from anterior (flexed) to posterior (extension) position.
Kinesio-taping of the coccyx to encourage coccyx extension.
Alignment of the sacrum using muscle energy techniques or mobilizations by a trained physical therapist.
TENS Unit for pain control
Foam rolling the gluts and sacrum. Be careful not to hurt the coccyx by rolling it over the foam roller.

Table 17.5: Medical Management of Coccydynia

MEDICAL MANAGEMENT OF COCCYDYNIA
Anti-inflammatory drugs (NSAIDs)
Steroidal injections
Surgery as *a last resort!!!*
Ganglion impar nerve block with or without coccygeal nerve
Muscle relaxers
Painkillers

External Manual Release and Exercises for the Relief of Coccyx Pain

The techniques and exercises highlighted in this section work on an overly flexed coccyx bone which is going into the anterior part of the body and is stuck or not moving properly. I am addressing this flexed position because most if not all the injuries that we see at my center are related to a flexed, stuck and/or deviated coccyx. I will also incorporate exercises to help release the coccyx that are safe and can be performed at any point. It is important to note here that the coccyx follows the lumbar spine. When the lumbar spine flexes, the coccyx bone also flexes and moves anteriorly. When the lumbar spine extends, the coccyx also extends and moves posteriorly. Sometimes my patients have so much pain that the only type of exercise they can do is this indirect exercise using the lumbar spine as a coupled mechanism to get the coccyx to move. Please clear all exercises with your MD. If you have coccyx pain and have experienced a fall or have just had a baby, make sure to rule out a fracture with an X-ray.

Butt Cheek Spread Hook

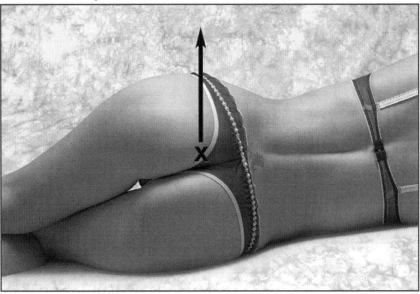

Description: Pull butt cheek in direction of arrow.

The butt cheek spread hook brings pain relief by working on the ligaments to the side of the coccyx bone. Not only does this technique help reduce fascial restrictions but it also helps to align a deviated side bent coccyx. When I use this technique with my patients and when I assign it to them as part of their self-care program, they rave about a reduction in their symptoms. If you find that your coccyx is deviated to one side focus on releasing that side only.

WHAT TO DO:

1. Lie on your right side and place the fingertips of the left hand on the side of your butt cheek at the gluteal cleft but as close to the coccyx as possible. Grip the area gently. You are gripping within the gluteal cleft into an area I call the coccyx crevice.

2. Exhale and pull the ligaments and fascia toward the top of the hip. Make sure to be in coccyx crevice and not on the fleshy gluteal muscles. The goal is to release fascial and ligament restrictions without pulling on the gluteal muscles.

3. Hold the outward stretch for 10 seconds and repeat 3 to 5 times. Switch sides and then repeat on the left side.

4. For an added release and to help the coccyx move from its stuck position couple this stretch with a reverse Kegel. As you perform the reverse Kegel imagine that your coccyx bone is moving from inside the body to the outside of the body.

External Massaging of the Coccyx Ligaments

Diagram 17.2: Posterior Coccyx Ligaments

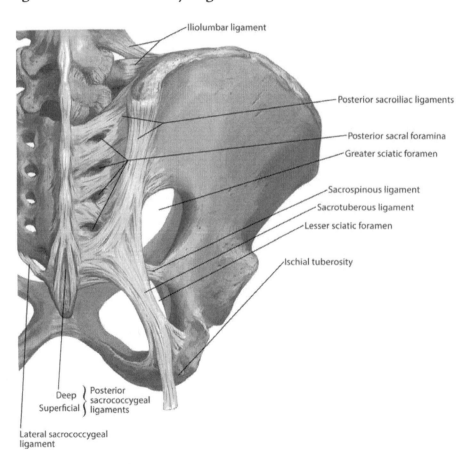

Description: For these next 2 techniques you will be working very close to the coccyx and massaging the coccygeal ligaments.

Source: Netter Images.

There are two great ways to massage the ligaments that have connections to the coccyx within the coccyx crevice space that is situated slightly below the gluteal cleft. In this small area you will have access to various ligaments that include sacrotuberous and sacrococcygeal. Many times these ligaments are painful and need gentle massaging in conjunction with the stretch from the butt cheek spread exercise. You will be performing longitudinal and cross friction massage strokes on these ligaments. This type of massaging should feel really great and bring relief. Some discomfort is expected but listen to your body; don't overdo it and don't dig in deep. Start superficially and as things improve you can massage more deeply.

WHAT TO DO:

1. Lie on your right side and place the left index finger below the gluteal cleft but inside the coccyx crevice. Use can use some oil if it's too painful to massage without it. I find lavender works well and it also helps to reduce spasms and quiet and relax the mind.

2. You will be performing two different types of strokes. The first stroke is an up-and-down stroke called longitudinal massage and the next stroke is a side stroke called cross friction massage. Cross friction tends to be more painful.

3. Massage the right side for up to 5 minutes and then move to the left side and repeat.

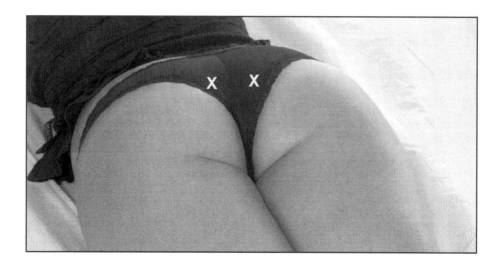

Double Cheek Spread with Movement

The "x" represents the location of the coccyx crevice

WHAT TO DO:

1. Lie on your stomach with a pillow under your chest and hips so that your head is over the pillow. This position will help to keep your neck in a neutral position. Your neck should be straight and you should be looking down. Don't drop the head and don't look up. Stay in neutral spine.

2. Place your fingertips in the coccyx crevice (as with the butt cheek spread exercise). Make sure your neck is comfortable and in neutral.

3. Exhale. Pull your fingertips in an outward direction and hold this stretch. Inhale as you are holding the stretch and simultaneously arch your back and point your toes inward and perform a reverse Kegel.

4. This is a super powerful exercise for the coccyx bone that couples a stretch and movement at the same time. Remember that the coccyx follows the lumbar spine and when you arch your lower back the coccyx moves from a flexed anterior position to an extended posterior position.

Stuck Drawer Technique for the Coccyx

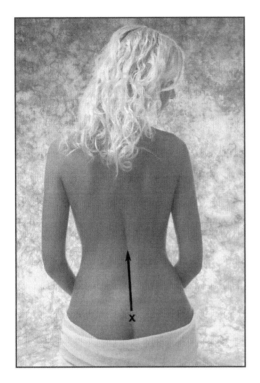

Place index finger on the "x" and pull upwards towards the head as stated below. This technique brings about remarkable results immediately and uses the PFMs to get the coccyx to move. It's very similar to the idea behind pulling a stuck drawer out. Sometimes when a drawer gets stuck you have to push it inward to get it to come out. It is ideal to have a physical therapist help you with this technique, but you will also achieve results working alone.

WHAT TO DO:

1. Sit upright in good sitting posture with your feet flat on the floor hip-width apart.

2. Place your right index finger at the aspect of the gluteal cleft at the sacro-coccygeal junction (where the "x" is on the photo). Make sure you have really good grip here because you will be tugging this area upward on the posterior sacrococcygeal ligament to get the coccyx to move.

3. As you are holding onto the sacrococcygeal ligaments and superior aspect of the coccyx bone, slump and flex your lumbar spine. In this position do a very gentle pelvic floor contraction, a Kegel. Hold for 10 seconds. Now get ready.

4. Exhale and simultaneously release the Kegel contraction (reverse Kegel), arch your back and pull upward on the sacrococcygeal ligaments.

5. Repeat 3 to 5 times. As you are releasing the Kegel you are bringing the coccyx back into its proper alignment with each repetition.

I also recommend that you see a physical therapist and have an internal mobilization of the coccyx. These mobilizations can be done vaginally or rectally. I find that many times patients with coccyx pain need a combination of therapies, and internal mobilization is one of them. Additional techniques to try from this book are foam rolling of the gluts and sacrum as highlighted in Chapter 8. You must also release any tension or spasms within the PFMs as they can pull the coccyx out of alignment and contribute to coccyx pain. Make sure to examine your PFMs and use the internal releasing techniques highlighted in Chapter 9.

In the next chapter we will cover intelligent core training for the restoration of female power and the relief of pelvic pain. There is much confusion when it comes to core training with pelvic pain so I will introduce you to the exercises that we successfully use at our healing center. I find that when we train the core the body is more able to withstand the stresses put upon it on a daily basis. Women also do much better with the therapy when the core is strong but not overly developed and engaged. I am a proponent of core training for function and pain relief. This is not a six-pack training routine but a lifelong program that offers exercises that will do you good even if you are 80 years old.

Chapter Eighteen

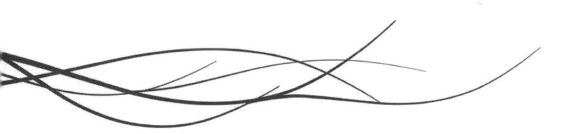

"It always seems impossible until it is done."

- Nelson Mandela

Chapter 18

THE NEW CORE FOR THE RESTORATION
OF FEMALE PELVIC POWER

Our abdominal muscles serve a far greater purpose than looking tight and awesome. This area is part of what I call the Pelvic Power relay station. The abdominal muscles create stability in our hips, PFMs and lumbar spine. Our midsections also provide support and stability for our internal organs, house the first two chakras and prevent energy leaks. If your abdominals are in a weakened state or are compromised by having a diastasis recti separation, you are at greater risk for female-related pelvic dysfunction. These problems include an increase in urinary leaking, urgency and frequency of urination, sexual dysfunction, abdominal trigger points, pelvic floor muscle weakness or spasms and pelvic/low back pain.

I cannot overstress the importance of intelligent core training. Many women love to work their abdominals, but are doing it all wrong by performing outdated exercises such as traditional crunches. Performing the same old crunches will not improve your female pelvic power. In fact, traditional abdominal exercises can actually be contributing to your female pelvic symptoms.

Women who have undergone abdominal surgeries, Cesarean births and myomectomies must really focus on properly re-training their core in order to prevent the incontinence, pelvic pain and muscle spasms that are so prevalent after surgery. For women with pelvic pain, the core is not something to be ignored. Women with pelvic pain are often told not to work on their abdominals because they risk having more pain. Sensible and intelligent core training will help women with both PFM weakness and PFM spasm.

The exercises in this chapter do not require that you put your hands behind your head and lift your shoulders off of the floor. Instead you will be working on the deepest abdominal muscle, the transversus abdominis, while simultaneously engaging your PFMs. This co-contraction creates power from within the body and can result in lifelong changes to your pelvic function. Proper co-contraction can result in improved sexual power, better bladder and bowel control, and less pelvic pain.

This co-contraction is a low-level gentle contraction of the PFMs and the transversus abdominis. Co-activation is not about gripping the PFMs nor is it about pulling in the abdominals with too much force. When you co-contract the PFMs and the transversus abdominis you do it at about 20 to 30 percent effort. This effort creates a root-lock mechanism, the kind all the yogis are talking about. The synergistic relationship of the PFMs and the abdominals is all about power and protection for your female parts. If you over-grip the transversus abdominis, you start to overactivate the other abdominal muscles such as the obliques; this is a big no-no. This is one of the reasons many traditional core programs fail. But my program succeeds because we first aim to correct the diastasis dysfunction and then we create core and pelvic power by strengthening without overactivating the PFMs (which could lead to more spasms and pain). Also remember that if you are over-gripping you will most likely start to hold your breath which creates an increase in intra-abdominal pressure —another no-no. Any increase in intra-ab-dominal pressure can lead to organ prolapse, increased leaking and PFM spasms. The New Core is all about conscious awareness, being fully present and not trying too hard to achieve the exercise.

This New Core should be performed by women when they have mastered the reverse Kegel exercise and are on the contract/relax Kegel program. I include this guideline here because I don't want you to experience more pelvic pain and spasms. At the bare minimum, you should close up the diastasis and work on training your transverse abdominal muscles. This is the way to start if you have progressed to the contract/relax Kegel program. Make sure to read and practice all the exercises in Chapter 4 before attempting the New Core for female pelvic power.

Now is the time to reclaim your body and to work within your fitness and symptom levels. First, I will describe what a diastasis recti separation is and how to test yourself for one. Then I will prescribe two corrective exercises to close up the separation and get you back on the road to reclaiming your pelvic power. The New Core Program includes eight levels, which can be found in Table 18.2. Before starting any of the exercises it is important to understand how to keep a neutral spine as most abdominal exercises will require this alignment. Practice neutral spine first and make sure you have it mastered and then embark on your journey to a more powerful core.

I have also included Table 18.3, which details the most common mistakes made while training the abdominal muscles using the New Core for Female Pelvic Power. Familiarize yourself with these common mistakes so that you don't repeat them as you progress in your core program. Once you have the proper foundation and your diastasis recti separation is closed up, you can then start on the New Core training for stronger abdominal muscles and lifelong female pelvic power. Now let's get started.

Specific Considerations for Abdominal Diastasis Recti Separation and the New Core Routine

Diastasis recti abdominis (DRA) is a separation of the rectus abdominis muscle at the linea alba. The outermost abdominal muscles, called the rectus abdominis, form two halves, called right and left recti muscles. These two halves are covered by fibrous connective tissue from other muscles and join at the central seam called the linea alba. Like a zipper, these abdominal muscles can separate due to incorrect biomechanics, pregnancy, with sudden weight gain and obesity. DRA can also result from performing abdominal exercises incorrectly or by suddenly sitting up straight in bed from a horizontal lying down position, called "jackknifing."

DRA has profound effects on the function of the pelvic floor muscles and bladder and bowel function. It is a well-known fact that the PFMs and the abdominals have a synergistic relationship. When DRA is present, it decreases the ability of the PFMs to contract effectively, contributing to urinary, stress and fecal incontinence and sexual dysfunction. DRA leaves the abdominals in a weakened state. When this separation is present in women with pelvic pain, the PFMs cannot function optimally, which makes the contract/relax exercises more difficult than they need to be. Make sure to test for DRA as defined in the next section. I would recommend not beginning the core series until your DRA measures two-fingers wide or less. Ideally I like the DRA to measure one-finger width as I find too much dysfunction with the PFMs when the separation is bigger.

It is also important to note that the function and insertion of the other abdominal muscles, called the transversus abdominis and internal/external obliques, are hindered when you have a DRA. This altered state of the abdominals can lead to the formation of trigger points in the abdominal wall. These abdominal trigger points can cause urinary urgency, pelvic pain and refer pain to the vulvar-vaginal area including the bladder. Many times these abdominal trigger points can lead to pain above the pubic bone and can cause the sensation of bladder infections without actually having one. Not only does the DRA need to be corrected, but also all of the abdominal trigger points need to be resolved in order to achieve symptom relief. Use the techniques outlined in Part III of this book to eliminate trigger points.

Before beginning the New Core program, you must first determine if you have a DRA by performing the test described below. If you find a DRA, perform the corrective exercises in order to close the gap before progressing to the more advanced core program. There are two exercises that you can perform to correct your DRA, one seated and one lying down on your back. If you have very weak abdominal muscles, start with the seated exercise and then incorporate the lying down corrective exercise in one week. It takes time to close up a DRA separation.

Closing a DRA requires that you are consistent with the exercises and that you consider the "Tips to Avoid Making the DRA Worse."

Diagram 18.1: Rectus Abdominus Muscles

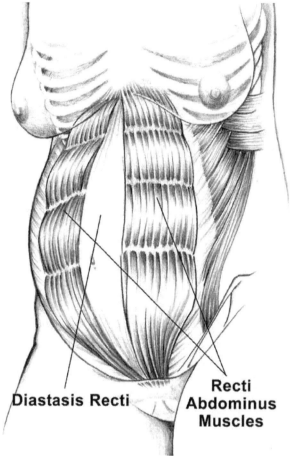

Source for Base Image: Winston Johnson

Tracking DRA Progress

It is important to track your DRA with a chart. It helps you to determine whether you need to increase the number of times you are doing the corrective exercise. I also think it's encouraging to see your progress as you do the hard work.

Table 18.1: DRA Tracking

Use this chart to keep track of your progress as you work to close your DRA.

DATE	2 INCHES ABOVE	AT UMBILICUS	2 INCHES BELOW

How to Test for DRA Separation

1. Lie on your back with your knees bent.

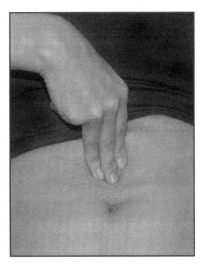

2. Exhale and slightly lift your upper back off the floor with your arms reaching forward. Check how many fingers you are able to insert horizontally two inches above the umbilicus, at the umbilicus, and two inches below the umbilicus.

3. DRA of one- to two-fingers separation is considered normal. A three-finger separation requires correction. Corrective exercises are used to close up any separation of the abdominals. The closer the DRA is

the less symptomatic you will be. If you still have symptoms at two-finger width, then you need to correct it first. DRA correction in my protocol is driven by symptoms, and for some women, the separation must be closed up to one-finger width. Always test at the same spots as indicated above. If you test at different spots your measurements will be inconsistent.

Tips to Avoid Making the DRA Worse

1. Avoid jackknifing out of bed. Instead, logroll out of bed by engaging your abdominals, turning completely to the side and then use your arms to push yourself to a seated position.

2. Avoid sudden weight gains.

3. Avoid yoga exercises that stretch the abdominals such as the Ball Wheel highlighted in Chapter 6.

4. Avoid coughing or sneezing without first engaging your abdominals.

5. Avoid traditional abdominal exercises such as abdominal crunches, which can make the DRA larger.

6. Avoid exercises at the gym or daily activities that make your belly pop out, also called the diastasis recti bulge.

7. Avoiding leaning forward such as bending from the hips to pick something up from the floor.

Finding Neutral Spine (NS)

Before we start with the corrective exercise for DRA, it is very important that you understand how to maintain and achieve neutral spine. Neutral spine is the natural position of the spine when all the parts of the spine, cervical, thoracic and lumbar, are in excellent alignment. This position is the most favorable when performing the New Female Pelvic Power Core program because in this position your abdominal and PFMs can optimally contract and relax as needed while executing the core program.

Neutral Spine (NS)

WHAT TO DO:

1. Lie on your back with your knees bent and your feet flat on the floor. Make sure your lower extremity is in great alignment. Imagine there is one continuous line from your hips to your knees to your feet. To accomplish this make sure your feet are parallel and not out to the side.

2. Keep your arms at your side and keep the body relaxed.

3. Exhale and use your abdominal muscles to press your lower back into the floor performing a posterior pelvic tilt (PPT). Inhale and release the PPT through your nose into your belly and release the PPT.

4. Exhale and pull your lower spine up and away from the floor creating an anterior pelvic tilt (ANT). Inhale and relax and release the ANT.

5. Most women have their spines either in an anterior pelvic tilt or a posterior pelvic tilt because of muscle imbalances and weakness. Neutral spine is a place in between these two extreme positions. You must practice this until you get a sense of what it means to be in neutral spine for you. Practice this exercise and know how to do it before moving forward.

Corrective DRA Exercises: Seated Splinted Holds

WHAT TO DO:

1. Sit in cross-legged position with correct posture, shoulders over hips.

2. Crisscross your hands over your belly, or use a scarf or Dyna-Band to bring the abdominals together.

3. Inhale through your nose into your belly. Exhale through your mouth to initiate the belly button reaching toward the spine, engaging the abdominals while keeping a NS. Hold this position.

4. Simultaneously, pull the sides of your abdominals together with your arms to approximate the recti muscles. You can also do a gentle PFM contraction while doing this exercise.

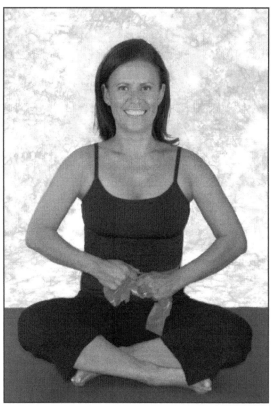

5. Breathe naturally and hold for five seconds. Return to start position.

6. Perform 20 times, two to three times a day.

Corrective DRA Exercises: Lying Down Splinted Head Raises

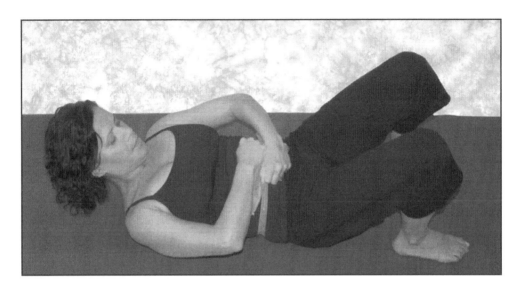

WHAT TO DO:

1. Lie on your back with your knees bent on the floor.

2. Bring your belly button gently to your spine while maintaining a NS.

3. Crisscross your hands over your belly, or use a scarf or Dyna-Band to bring the abdominals together.

4. Exhale very slowly, contract your abdominals and raise your head toward your chest just before the diastasis bulge begins. To begin, keep the shoulders in contact with the floor. To maximize the approximation of the recti muscles you can use a large scarf or wrap to bring the muscles together. You should also do a gentle PFM contraction while doing this exercise.

5. Breathe naturally and hold for five seconds. Return to start position. As you get stronger, you will be able to lift your shoulders off the floor.

6. Perform 20 times, two to three times a day.

Once you have become aware of your diastasis and have begun to take corrective measures, you will be ready to move ahead into the Pilates series in Chapter 5 and the New Core for Female Pelvic Power abdominal exercises described below.

Your Diastasis Recti Is Corrected: What Now?

Once you have corrected your diastasis recti and it is within a one to two-finger separation, you are now ready to embark on the more difficult core exercises of the Female Pelvic Power Program. All of the exercises in this amazing program involve a transverse belly hold. You must master this foundational exercise first, before progressing through the rest of the New Core program.

How to Progress in the Abdominal Program

There are several exercises to the New Core program for female pelvic power. It is important not to move to a more difficult exercise before you master the previous level. When you can perform 20 reps, two to three times in great form you have mastered that level and can move to the next level. You can be working at two levels at the same time on different exercises as long as you have mastered the previous level.

Table 18.2: The New Core for Female Pelvic Power

NAME OF TECHNIQUE
Corrective DRA Exercises, Seated or Lying Down Level 1
Transverse Belly Holds: Foundational exercise for all other exercises: Level 1
Leg Press: Level 2
Marching: Level 3
Up-Up/Down-Down: Level 4
Toe Taps: Level 5
Bicycles: Level 6
Planks: Level 7
Side Planks: Level 8

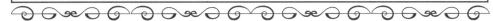

Table 18.3: Common Mistakes: What to Avoid in Your Female Pelvic Power Training Program

COMMON MISTAKES: WHAT TO AVOID IN YOUR FEMALE PELVIC POWER TRAINING PROGRAM
1. Avoid holding your breath while performing your abdominal exercises. If you hold the breath, you could leak urine, push the organs downward, create PFMs spasms and not activate the core muscles correctly.
2. Do not advance to a more difficult abdominal exercise without first mastering the previous level.
3. Never leak urine. If you leak with your abdominal exercises, then the exercise is too difficult for you. You should return to the previous level and master those exercises without leaking.
4. Do not exacerbate your pelvic pain. There is a thin line between intelligent working out and creating more tension in the abdominal and PFMs. If you experience an increase in pain, you should return to the previous level and master those exercises without pain.
5. Avoid sticking your butt into the air when performing exercises such as plank. If you find that you are sticking out your butt, then you are using too much of your arm and leg power.
6. Do not flare out your ribs when doing the core program. Instead keep them pulled in toward your navel. If your ribs pop out, then you are not activating the core properly.
7. Avoid sagging the lower back when performing your plank exercises.
8. Do not over-contract your abdominal core muscles. Over-contraction activates the obliques instead of the deeper transversus abdominis muscle. You are over-contracting if you feel a bearing-down sensation in the pelvis or if your lower abdominals "pop out" with contraction. You may also feel increased pelvic pressure if you overactivate the abdominal core muscles.
9. Do not forget to co-contract the PFMs with the transverse holds while performing the New Core exercises. True core strength requires activation of both muscle groups through the entire set of exercises. This co-contraction is at about 20 to 30 percent of effort, not 100 percent. Remember: PFM is a low-level contraction.
10. Avoid rounding or arching the lower back while performing the core exercises. Keep your spine in neutral while performing all the exercises.

Transverse Belly Holds

WHAT TO DO:

1. This exercise may be done sitting, supine or standing. Keep a neutral spine as you take a full belly breath. As you exhale draw your belly closer and more firmly toward the spine. As you pull in your abdominals try to imagine that you are trying to squeeze into an old pair of jeans that don't fit. Make sure to keep a NS.

2. Additional cues that work well to activate and train the transverse muscle are:

   a. Imagine that you are doing a Kegel that moves all the way up to the lower part of your abdominals.

   b. Imagine that there is a guy wire from the right anterior hip bone to the left and imagine the guy wire becoming slack as you bring the two hip bones together.

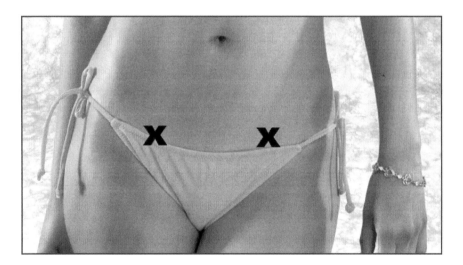

3. Once you establish the above movement, hold for five seconds and repeat ten times. Do one to three sets per day. Use the different cues to help you. Although this exercise looks easy it is extremely difficult to train and isolate the transverse muscle. This exercise is the building block for all the exercises that follow so take your time and practice it.

WHAT TO WATCH OUT FOR:

1. Holding the breath, which can increase leaking or pelvic pain.

2. Over-contracting the abdominals, which engages the more superficial abdominals, such as the rectus abdominis and external obliques.

3. Increased abdominal pain or trigger points in the abdominals and/or an increase in your symptoms.

Leg Press

WHAT TO DO:

1. Lie flat on the floor with your lower back in neutral spine and rest your arms on the side. Engage your transversus abdominis and your PFMs. Keep this engagement at 20 to 30 percent of effort.

2. Hug your knees into your chest, then release your knees slightly away from you until they form a 90 degree angle.

3. Bring your outstretched hand or hands to your thighs and gently push your hands into your thighs making sure your legs don't move. Continue this pressing into your thighs for five seconds and then rest. Repeat ten times or as tolerated.

4. You may also try this in a seated position with your feet flat on the floor. This is a great exercise to do at work.

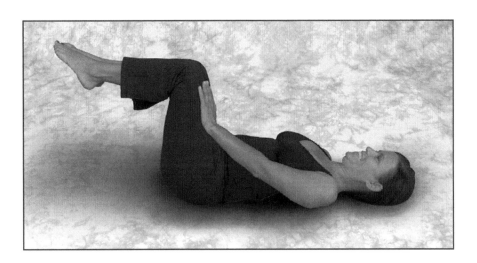

WHAT TO WATCH OUT FOR:

1. Moving the legs and pressing too hard. This exercise is a sustained hold with no movement.

2. Holding the breath. Breathe naturally as you hold the resistance against your thighs.

3. Allowing the rectus abdominis to "pop out" during the exercise. If your belly bulges or your back comes off the floor, then you have likely lost your transverse belly hold and the NS.

Marching

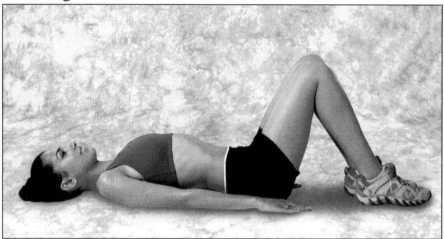

WHAT TO DO:

1. Lie flat on the floor with a NS and rest your arms on the side. Engage your transversus abdominis and your PFMs. Keep this engagement at 20 to 30 percent of effort.

2. Slowly raise the right leg one to three inches from the floor. Keep trunk rigid. Hold three seconds. Lower the right leg and then slowly raise the left leg one to three inches from the floor. Keep trunk rigid. Hold for three seconds.

3. Repeat ten times on each leg.

4. Remember to keep the hips still and stable while performing this exercise. Do not move back and forth as you switch legs.

WHAT TO WATCH OUT FOR:

1. Holding the breath, which can increase leaking or pelvic pain.

2. Over-contracting, which engages the more superficial abdominals, such as the rectus abdominis and external obliques.

3. Moving the pelvis and trunk and lifting the legs too high off the floor.

Up-Up/Down-Down

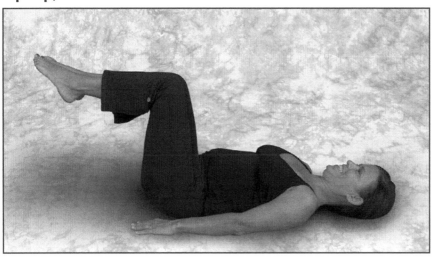

WHAT TO DO:

1. Lie flat on the floor with a NS and rest your arms on the side. Engage your transversus abdominis and your PFMs. Keep this engagement at 20 to 30 percent of effort.

2. Hug your knees into your chest, then release your knees slightly away from you until they form a 90 degree angle.

3. Holding the trunk stable and maintaining a transverse belly hold, release the right knee slightly away from you, then release the left to meet the right. This is the "down-down" position.

4. Then draw the right knee back up to 90 degrees followed by the left. This is the "up-up" position.

5. Continue in this down-down, up-up movement pattern for 20 reps. Maintain NS throughout the exercise. Repeat eight to ten times with the goal of reaching 20 reps.

WHAT TO WATCH OUT FOR:

1. Holding the breath, which can increase leaking or pelvic pain.

2. Over-contracting, which engages the more superficial abdominals, such as the rectus abdominis and external obliques.

3. The down-down position is the hardest position. Avoid arching your back, as this can cause a strain or injury to the lower back.

Toe Taps

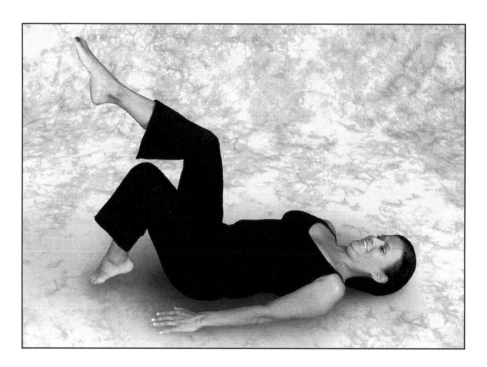

WHAT TO DO:

1. Lie flat on the floor with a NS and rest your arms on the side. Engage your transverse abdominal muscles and your PFMs. Keep this engagement at 20 to 30 percent of effort.

2. Start by hugging your knees into your chest, then release your knees slightly away from you until they form a 90 degree angle.

3. Slowly lower right leg toward the floor (keep your knees bent to tap your toes to the floor). Once you tap the right toe, raise your leg back up to the start position. Then lower your left leg until the toe touches the floor or mat. Once you tap the left toe, raise your leg back up to the start position.

4. Continue in this pattern of right toe touch, back to start position and then left toe touch for 20 reps. Repeat for two to three sets or as tolerated.

WHAT TO WATCH OUT FOR:

1. Holding the breath, which can increase leaking, pelvic pressure or pelvic pain.

2. Performing the toe taps too quickly, which will hinder the effectiveness of this exercise. Focus on performing the exercise correctly, with a transverse belly hold and minimal rocking of the pelvis.

3. Avoid arching your lower back, as this can cause a strain or injury to the lower back.

4. Moving the pelvis and hips too much and doing the exercise too quickly.

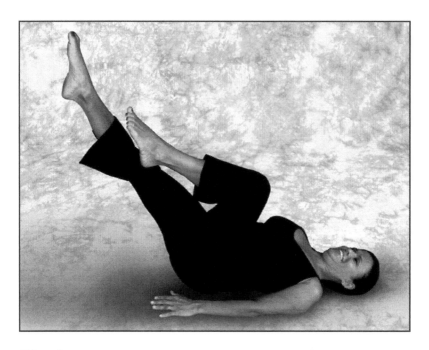

Bicycles

WHAT TO DO:

1. Lie flat on the floor with a NS and rest your arms on the side. Engage your transversus abdominis and your PFMs. Keep this engagement at 20 to 30 percent of effort.

2. Bring your knees up to about a 90 degree angle and slowly go through a bicycle pedal motion as pictured. This should be a smooth and fluid motion as if you are riding a bicycle. Keep the legs high. The lower your legs are the more difficult this exercise becomes. It is best to start with a high bicycle and then lower the legs when you are super strong.

3. Perform the exercise in a slow, controlled motion. Repeat 10 to 20 times on each side.

WHAT TO WATCH OUT FOR:

1. Performing the exercise too quickly and losing the form and control.

2. Avoid arching your low back, as this can cause a strain or injury to the lower back muscles, which help stabilize the core.

3. Performing the bicycle with the legs too low, which is very difficult when you are not ready to do so. Be careful not to injure your back and create spasms in the PFMs.

Planks

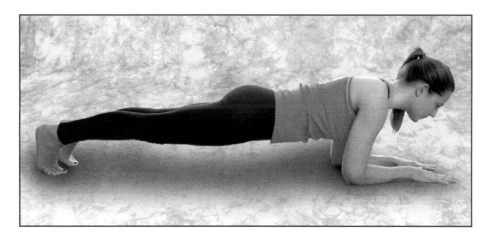

WHAT TO DO:

1. Get into push-up position on the floor. Now bend your elbows 90 degrees and rest your weight on your forearms. Your elbows should be directly beneath your shoulders, and your body should form a straight line from your head to your feet.

2. Hold the plank position for ten seconds or as tolerated. The goal here would be 60-second holds. Repeat five to ten times. If this exercise is too difficult make it easier by placing your knees on the floor. Remember to lift the feet off the floor for this easier version. (Note: This version of the exercise is not shown in the photograph.)

WHAT TO WATCH OUT FOR:

1. Keep your spine straight and do not stick your butt into the air.

2. Avoid arching your low back, as this can cause a strain or injury to the lower back. Keep your spine in neutral.

Side Planks

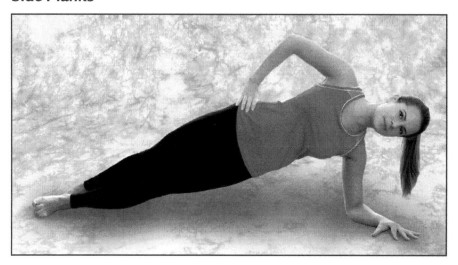

WHAT TO DO:

1. Lie on your side on the mat. Place your forearm on the mat, directly under and perpendicular to your body. Place your upper leg directly on top of your lower leg and straighten your knees and hips.

2. Raise your body upward by straightening the waist, so that your body is stable and rigid. Hold position. Repeat with opposite side.

3. Hold the side plank position for ten seconds or as tolerated. Repeat five to ten times.

WHAT TO WATCH OUT FOR:

1. Keep position straight and do not sag in the middle of the body.

2. Breathe naturally.

3. Make sure the DRA is closed. Side planks can open the DRA so always test your DRA to make sure you haven't reopened it with this exercise.

Now that our foundation is almost set, let's build upon this and examine our bladders in more detail. Chapter 13 discusses the bladder but in the next chapter I give you additional tools that, when incorporated into your healing program, will bring great results. Make sure to go back and re-read Chapter 13 before progressing to Chapter 19. Together both chapters will teach you how to tame and control your bladder and your symptoms. So read on...

Chapter Nineteen

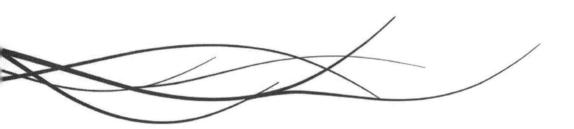

"Let me not pray to be sheltered from dangers, but to be fearless in facing them. Let me not beg for the stilling of my pain, but for the heart to conquer it."
- Rabindranath Tagore

Chapter 19

THE REAL DEAL: HOW TO HEAL YOUR BLADDER

In this chapter I will discuss how to manage your bladder and get it back under your control. I am going to share with you "real deal" bladder information that will consist of massage, foam rolling, and helpful tips that will put your bladder back on track. This discussion builds on the Better Bathroom Habits chapter so use it as a reference as you go through this chapter. It may come as a surprise to you but your bladder pain could be coming from somewhere else within your body. The bladder is one of those organs with many connections to different parts of the body. These connections occur via fascia, nerve and muscle. This chapter will help you explore your body so that you can find these body parts that are referring pain, urgency and frequency to your bladder. The bladder also has a deep connection to the anterior wall of the pelvic floor muscles; you will have to investigate that area of the PFMs in a gentle and thorough manner.

Your bladder should hold about 300 to 500 ml of urine, which correlates to about 10 to 16 ounces. When the bladder is full it sends a message to your brain telling it that it is ready to be emptied. When you void you should empty to a very low volume and there should be no feelings of incomplete emptying. Experiencing these symptoms is an indicator that your bladder needs work and training and that there is also a dysfunction within the PFMs. Additionally there should never be pain, urge, post-dribble leaking or a need to push the urine out with voiding. This may surprise many readers because these behaviors and symptoms have become so natural to you that you may have forgotten what a normal void feels and looks like. But these voiding patterns are dysfunctional and if not corrected will create havoc and misery in your life. Remember that the bladder and the PFMs talk to each other, so if the bladder decides to behave badly, the PFMs will also start to misbehave. For the bladder to empty completely the PFMs need to be able to relax and let go. If the PFMs have trigger points, spasms and/or poor coordination then there is a higher risk for bladder dysfunction. Conversely, when the PFMs relax the bladder contracts, but if the bladder starts to contract or spasm inappropriately or at the wrong times then that can lead to urge, leaking with urge and an increase in frequency. Before you know it you have become a slave to your bladder and you are looking for a bathroom everywhere you go. Urge leakage can happen at any time, but many of my patients report that it occurs around a certain activity. For instance many of my patients complain of "key in the door" syndrome: they start to get the urge and leak as they open the doors to their houses. This experience is common and can be put under control with some of the urge techniques highlighted in Table 19.1.

Now let's start to learn what will bring resolution to your bladder pain, frequency and urge symptoms. Start out slowly and methodically and try all the techniques and then focus on the ones that give you the most relief. At first you will be very challenged but with time the trade secrets I am about to share will enable you to resolve many of your bladder issues.

The Successful Bladder: What You Need to Know Now

Urge Control

Urge control and suppression techniques are important because they not only buy you time to get to the toilet dry but they also help to retrain the bladder back to health. This will take time so don't become discouraged if at first you can't beat your urge; with time and practice you will.

TABLE 19.1: Urge Control Techniques

URGE CONTROL TECHNIQUES
Cross your legs and put pressure on the urethra when the urge hits. This will buy you some time.
Perform a quick Kegel contraction. Start with 10 and continue until the urge has subsided. Be careful not to go into PFM spasms.
Apply pressure on the perineum or clitoris.
Slow down your pace and move slowly. Do not rush or run to the bathroom.
Begin deep diaphragmatic breathing and continue breathing this way until the urge subsides.
Distract your mind from the urge. Occupy yourself with another activity or think of something else.
Tighten your gluteal muscles and curl your toes under. This helps to shut down the nerves that innervate the bladder.
Keep your body as warm as possible. Cold stimulates the bladder.
Don't slouch; keep your body upright and arch your back slightly to reduce pressure on the bladder.
Loosen your pants or shirt tops to reduce pressure on the bladder.

Avoid "Just in Case" Urination: The JIC Stops Now

Many women suffer from dysfunctional voiding patterns because we are urinating out of habit and not waiting for the bladder to fill and to get the normal urge that comes from a full bladder. A normal bladder empties 6 to 8 times a day with about 3 to 4 hour intervals in between each void. This is the desired interval and frequency, but for many women this might not be possible. So what should you do? Listen to your bladder and achieve the best that you can for you. Even if that means that you are voiding more often. Remember that every time we go to the bathroom "just in case" we disrupt the normal rhythm of the bladder.

It is difficult to override habits and easy to continue doing the same thing over and over again. But the bladder can be finicky and temperamental so it is important to eliminate all "just in case" voids from your life. This is the only way to a peaceful and happy bladder. To succeed here you have to track your bladder patterns to see if you are having any JIC voids.

Sex and Urinary Tract Infections (UTI)

For many women sex is a trigger for bladder infections. It is important for them to urinate before and after sex as a preventive measure. Many of the women I treat also take an antibiotic after sex to prevent infections. These patients believe in this preventive measure and it works for them, but a good probiotic should be part of this preventive care as well. What you will find is that after you tame your bladder and normalize your PFMs you might not need to continue the antibiotic or you can cut back.

Public Bathrooms and Bad Bladder Habits

Women often tell me they are unable to sit in public restrooms so they squat/hover over the toilet instead. This type of squatting is bad news for your bladder. Your PFMs and leg muscles contract when you squat making it difficult if not impossible to urinate properly without pushing. It is my recommendation that you sit on the toilet in public restrooms. You can always place a protective covering or toilet paper on the seat.

Your Bladder Is What You Eat and Drink: Healthy Bladder Habits

Your bladder responds to your diet and fluid intake. The bladder is a reactive organ and communicates "loud and clear" to you. Many women come to my healing center, Renew Physical Therapy, in a state of extreme dehydration. Their rationale is: "If I drink less, I will pee less and I will go to the bathroom fewer times." This is an incorrect assumption. The less you drink the more your urine becomes concentrated and the more irritated the bladder becomes. Drink water and keep your urine a pale yellow color; this will decrease your bladder's reactivity and you will be able to train the bladder more easily when it's calm and happy.

Carbonated Water and Drinks Are Bad News for the Bladder

A while back I was evaluating the bladder diary of a patient. (Please see Chapter 13 to acquaint yourself with this life-saving tool.) This patient was urinating over 25 times a day. She was despondent and had urgency all the time and was leaking. She told me she drank water all day long. Her diary showed that what she actually drank was carbonated water with lemon. I immediately told her to eliminate the carbonated water and to switch to regular water without lemon. This simple change in her diet helped to restore normal bladder function. This was an easy case, but it demonstrates the importance of hydration with regular water.

If you drink more water, you will not pee more but less. Monitor your water intake and drink throughout the day. Don't guzzle a lot of water at a single time. It might also be helpful to have your last glass of water by 8 or 9 PM to eliminate getting out of bed at night to urinate.

Seeing Is Believing

Sometimes when we are at our deepest suffering we forget to check in with ourselves and take a good look at our habits. A bladder diary is key if you are to retrain and control your bladder again. Please take a look at Chapter 13 and start to keep a bladder diary. I recommend that you keep one for one day during the week and for one day during the weekend. We behave differently when we are away from the stresses of our jobs. This diary will paint a picture for you and you will get the clarity and the information that you need to retrain your bladder. The bladder is an easy organ to take control over but you have to be diligent and relentless. Start right away. You may have to keep this diary for several weeks because it is just as important to track your progress and to determine how and when to increase your voiding intervals.

Table 19.2: Daily Voiding Diary

TIME OF DAY	FOOD/LIQUID (OTHER THAN WATER) INTAKE: STATE TYPE OF FOOD AND DRINK	WATER INTAKE (OUNCES)	AMOUNT URINATED (COUNTED IN "MISSIS-SIPPIS")	URGE PRESENT (LOW, MEDIUM OR HIGH) LEAKING? (Y/N?) IF YES, WHAT WERE YOU DOING?
6AM				
7AM				
8AM				
9AM				
10AM				
11AM				
12PM				
1PM				
2PM				
3PM				
4PM				
5PM				
6PM				
7PM				
8PM				
9PM				
10PM				
11PM				
12AM				
Overnight				

PDF version of this table available at *http://www.RenewPT.com.*

Watch What You Eat

There are so many foods that can upset the bladder that the list is endless. I touch upon this in Chapter 13. The goal is to track which foods are making your bladder reactive and cut them out until you have control over your symptoms. Of course there are common foods like citrus, chocolate, tomatoes, wine, beer, artificial sweeteners, sodas, caffeine and fruit juices that wreak havoc on the bladder, but you really need to see what affects your bladder and gives you urgency, frequency and/or pain. Some women may do well with tomatoes and others will not. You have to discover these nuances by keeping track of your food and fluid intake and then determine what ticks off your bladder. Please use the bladder diary in Chapter 13 to track your food, fluid and progress. For more information on this topic, visit Jill Osborne's website *www.IC-Network.com.*

Hands-On Techniques for Better Bladder Health

Trigger Points for Urgency, Frequency and Bladder Pain Outside the Bladder

If I had a dollar for every time that I found bladder urge and pain stemming from the muscles of the legs, butt, or abdominal area, I would have a lot of money. In this section I will cover the body parts that you need to investigate for bladder symptoms. I will also give you several amazing exercises and tools that will help you to resolve your bladder dysfunction. The areas of interest here are the inner thigh muscles, the suprapubic abdominal muscles and the sacrum. Many times these areas are loaded with trigger points that are referring to the bladder; you have to resolve these trigger points to get the bladder back under control.

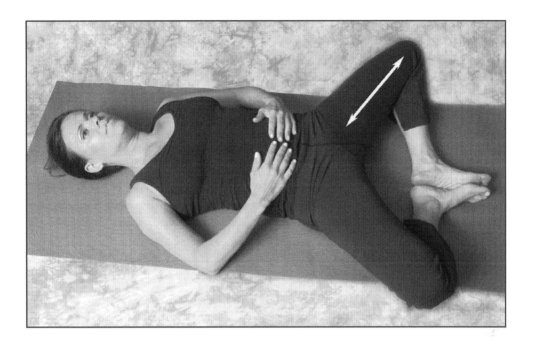

Inner Thigh Trigger Point Release

GETTING STARTED:

This external technique is repeated from Chapter 10 because spasms and pain in the inner thigh muscles have a direct connection to the bladder and PFMs, and require special attention. The inner thigh muscles can develop spasms, trigger points and adhesions in them as a response to what is happening internally in the bladder. These tissue abnormalities can lead to bladder urgency and pain. The trigger points in the inner thigh can refer to the bladder. A trigger point will feel like a hard, small ball and will produce pain when touched. In terms of the bladder a trigger point in this area may also give you urge.

WHAT TO DO:

1. Examine your inner thigh muscles by sweeping your hands over them. You are searching for trigger points, spasms or areas that give your bladder

symptoms.

2. Once you find them, press into the trigger points for 90 seconds until the pain has diminished or gone away. You may have to do several cycles of 90 seconds to accomplish this.

3. Complete normalization of the inner thigh is necessary because this muscle is a major culprit in creating bladder symptoms such as urgency and bladder pain.

Foam Roller Inner Thigh/Groin

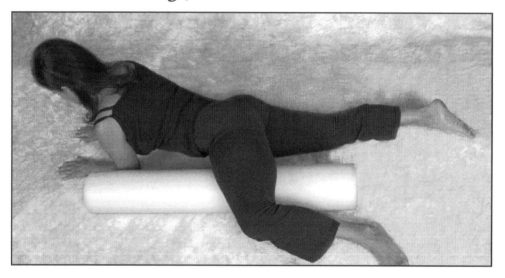

It is important to complement your trigger point work on the inner thighs with foam rolling. The rolling will help to normalize tension and spasms within the inner thighs.

WHAT TO DO:

1. Balance on your elbows and place the foam roller on the right inner thigh by flexing the right hip to the side and bending the knee. You may have to move your hands for better rolling. Your elbows should both be on one side of the roller.

2. Slowly roll from the top of the groin to the knee.

3. Break up the rolling into the upper groin, the middle inner thigh and the lower thigh area for better emphasis. Avoid rolling over the knee joint.

4. Roll 1 to 2 minutes over your inner thighs. Focus on the painful spots and concentrate the rolling and rocking on the areas where you find pain and restrictions.

5. Switch legs and repeat on the other side.

Suprapubic External Bladder Trigger Points

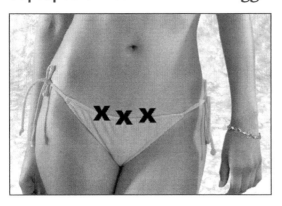

Many of my patients complain about pain right above the pubic bone. The bladder lives underneath this bone. It makes sense that if there is a dysfunction in the bladder that the top of the pubic bone and the lower abdominal area will be painful and filled with trigger points. This technique brings about amazing results and can help reduce bladder urgency. Many times trigger points in this area refer pain to the bladder. This is one of my go-to techniques for women suffering from bladder conditions.

WHAT TO DO:

1. Start your investigation by pressing along the top of the pubic bone and your lower abdominal muscle area. Take note of where the pain is and what symptoms you feel when you press into these areas.

2. Make yourself a simple map. Note pain level from 0 to 10 (0 = no pain, 10 = worst pain) and symptoms produced.

3. Hold the trigger point for 90 seconds, making sure to release the trigger point slowly. Repeat as many times as necessary until the pain level is reduced by 50 percent or you feel relief from the symptoms.

4. CAUTION: Do not press into an area that has a pulse. If you feel a pulse, move to a different area.

Massage and Connective Tissue Release Techniques for the Relief of Bladder Symptoms

Psoas Release

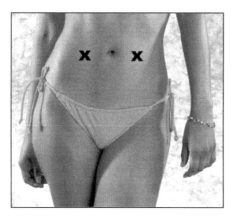

Your body has two very deep muscles on either side of the lower abdomen called the psoas muscles. These muscles attach from the lower spine to the hip bones, and help flex the hips. The psoas muscles are frequently very painful, in spasm, and irritated in women suffering from pelvic pain. The kidneys have an intimate connection to this muscle. Keeping the psoas muscle pain free, supple and flexible is critical. This technique is highly effective in reducing bladder pain and urgency, improving bladder function and reducing pelvic pain symptoms.

WHAT TO DO:

1. Lie on your back with your legs straight out.

2. Go about two to three inches to the right side of your belly button. Place your fingertips into the area, slowly allowing them to sink into your abdomen and being careful to avoid any feelings of an artery pulse.

3. Lift your right leg straight up and you will feel the psoas pop into your hand. It may take a little practice to get this but keep trying. Once you know where the psoas muscle is, place your fingertips in that spot and slowly press downward into the psoas for 60 to 90 seconds. If you feel any tingling, numbness, or tremendous increase in pain, get off the area and try to relocate the psoas muscle. Switch sides and do the left psoas muscle release.

4. CAUTION: Do not press into an area that has a pulse. If you feel a pulse, move to a different area and locate the muscle at another place.

Bladder Up-Glide Massage

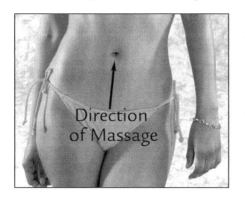

Direction of Massage

There are three ligaments that arise from the umbilicus like a tripod and attach to the superior aspect of the bladder. These ligaments are called collectively the urachus ligaments. They have to function well and help with the upward movement that the bladder undergoes when it fills. Massaging this ligamentous area is important for bladder health and function.

WHAT TO DO:

1. Place your fingertips on the top of your pubic bone and massage upward toward the belly button.

2. Maintain firm but gentle pressure as you massage upward.

3. Repeat for 30 strokes. If you discover a trigger point along the way make sure to take care of it by pressing into the trigger point for 60 to 90 seconds.

Eliminating Urge and Bladder Dysfunction with Internal PFM Methods

Quite frequently I find that urge and bladder pain come from the PFMs. PFMs refer bladder symptoms because they are connected to the bladder via fascia, nerves and blood supply. The bladder is supported and housed by the anterior wall of the PFMs. So a dysfunction in the bladder many times correlates to trigger points, spasms and inflexible anterior wall PFMs. Accessing this wall can be difficult and I often recommend that a Crystal Wand be used. I prefer that initially you use your fingers to get to the anterior wall of PFMs. This can easily be performed while sitting on the toilet and inserting the finger up to the second layer. Once in the second layer turn the finger upward in a "come hither" shape so that the tip of the finger is pointing to the PFMs that live under the pubic bone on the anterior wall. You can use a Crystal Wand but you must be careful not to press too hard on these muscles as they are delicate and you can hurt yourself. Now let's go back to the PFMs clock. You will be working at the 2 o'clock position on the left and the 10 o'clock position on the right. NEVER press directly onto the 12 o'clock position because this is where your bladder lives.

WHAT TO DO:

1. Find a comfortable position that gives you easy access to the anterior wall of the PFMs.

2. Imagine the PFM clock and locate your 10 and 2 o'clock positions. This is where you will focus your work.

3. Place your finger into the vagina with plenty of lubricant and turn your hand upward so that your finger can access the 10 o'clock position on the right.

4. Feel around this area and search for areas within the muscle that reproduce your urge and/or bladder symptoms. Using the trigger point release therapy press into this area until your urge or pain has subsided by more than 50 percent or is eliminated altogether.

5. Now move to the 2 o'clock position and search for spots in the muscle that cause your symptoms.

6. Remember to avoid the 12 o'clock position and do not get off the trigger points until the symptoms have subsided by more than 50 percent. If you don't shut down these trigger points you will have more urge, more pain and possible leaking.

Normalize Your PFMs with the Reverse Kegel

As previously discussed the bladder and PFMs are intimately connected. Remember that you must focus on all the muscle parts of your PFMs to get them normalized and working properly. It is critical to master not only reverse Kegels but to eventually get the PFMs on a contract/relax program. The reverse Kegel allows for the initiation of urination and defecation and must be mastered to get the bladder and bowels under control. At first the reverse Kegel can be difficult to accomplish but please refer to Chapter 4 because it will help you achieve mastery of this exercise. The guidelines in Chapter 4 are instrumental in helping you to get back on track with your urinary function. To normalize tension, remove trigger points and to stretch your PFMs follow the guidelines in Chapter 9. Normalizing the PFMs takes hard work and dedication. Set-backs will be encountered but the secret to life is to fall seven times but get up eight.

Conclusion

You've done it! You've gone all the way through my book. If this is your first read, take the time to re-read, review and begin to absorb the nuances as you experiment with crafting your program from your new sets of tools. Armed with information and determination, embark on your journey to relieving your pain and don't look back. Please check out my website, *www.RenewPT.com,* for the most current information. I am always adding new material to my great site and invite you to get involved in spreading the word to women who have suffered long enough. I invite you to become the heroine of your own story.

Appendices, Glossary Bibliography, and Index

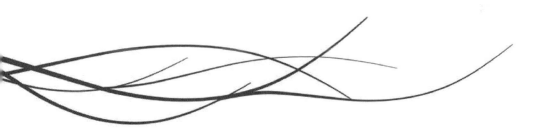

*"The course of our lives is determined by how we react—
what we decide and what to do—at the darkest times.
The nature of that response determines a
person's true worth and greatness."*

—Daisaku Ikeda

Appendix 1

Essential Oil Resources

Medical Disclaimer:

The essential oil information listed below is for educational purposes only and not a substitute for healthcare or medical advice. You must check with your doctor, caregiver and/or oncologist before working with essential oils. It is advisable to seek help from a trained aromatherapist when working with oils. There are also custom oil blends available in our store at *www.RenewPT.com*.

Essential Oils for Chronic Pain:

- Helichrysum Essential Oil
- Peppermint Essential Oil
- Wintergreen Essential Oil
- Oregano Essential Oil
- Balsam Fir Essential Oil
- Marjoram Essential Oil

Essential Oils for Muscle Pain:

- Roman Chamomile Essential Oil
- Peppermint Essential Oil
- Rosemary Essential Oil
- Thyme Essential Oil
- Wintergreen Essential Oil
- Marjoram Essential Oil
- Basil Essential Oil

Essential Oils for Bladder Health:

- Lavender Essential Oil
- Tea Tree Essential Oil
- Oregano Essential Oil

Renew PT Custom Oil Blends:

- Blues Fighter
- Down There Oil Vaginal Serum
- Sacred Renewal Spray
- SOS Scar Care Oil

The information listed above is cited from *Essential Oils Integrative Medical Guide* by Gary Young, Essential Science Publishing (2003).

Appendix 2

Resources

Renew Physical Therapy Website

www.RenewPT.com. Free information, blank pdfs of EFP book charts for your pain mapping, pain journaling, DRA testing, Q-Tip test, voiding diary, custom oil blends for pelvic pain, blogs, research, and other important tools. Also published case study on scar therapy at Renew PT, *http://tinyurl.com/kfllqrw.*

American College of Obstetricians and Gynecologists. Resource Guide *www. acog.org.*

American Physical Therapy Association. 1-800-999-APTA. Physical Therapy for the pelvic floor- Select Women's Health. *www.APTA.org.*

The Business of Being Born. Great information for all women planning to have a baby. *www.thebusinessofbeingborn.com.*

Dilator Sets. Available on this site. *www.vaginismus.com.*

Endometriosis Association. *www.endometriosisassn.org.*

Herbal and Flower Products. For vaginal steams and penal washes. *www.mountainroseherbs.com.*

Holly Herman & Kathe Wallace. Best teachers in pelvic floor rehab. Call to get a recommendation for a pelvic floor rehab specialist. Telephone - 646-355-8777. *http://hermanwallace.com.*

Menopause Society of North America. *www.menopause.org*

Interstitial Cystitis Network. *www.IC-network.org.*

Interstitial Cystitis Association. *www.IChelp.org.*

International Cesaerian Awareness Network. *www.ICAN-online.org.*

International Society for the Study of Vulvovaginal Disease. *www.issvd.org.*

IPPS: The International Pelvic Pain Society. *www.PelvicPain.org.*

Midwives Alliance of North America. *www.mana.org.*

My Best Birth. Ricki Lake and Abby Epstein's great resource for women. *www.mybestbirth.com.*

National Fibromyalgia Association. *www.fmaware.org.*

NVA: National Vulvodynia Association. *www.NVA.org.*

Vulvodynia Online Resource. *www.vulvodynia.com.*

Water Based Lubricant. *www.slipperystufflubes.com*

Young Living Essential Oils

Website: *www.youngliving.com/en_US/.* For medical/therapeutic grade essential oils, shop at Young Living. This is the brand I trust the most. Please use my subscriber number ID #1422496 to get a wholesale membership. There is a small membership enrollment fee to buy oils at wholesale that ranges from $40 to $275.

Glossary

Adhesions. Fibrous bands that form between tissues and organs as a result of the healing process that occurs after surgical procedures, inflammation, trauma or infection.

Alcock's Canal. A structure within the pelvis through which the pudendal nerve, internal pudendal artery and internal pudendal veins travel. This structure is like a canal formed by the obturator internus fascia.

Anal Rim. The sensitive tissue surrounding the anal sphincter. This area can become very painful when there are spasms of the pelvic floor muscles and the muscles of the anal sphincter.

Anismus. A malfunction of the external anal sphincter and puborectalis (part of the PFM) muscle during defecation. Failure of these muscles to relax during defecation causes obstructed defecation and constipation.

Bartholin's Glands. Glands located to the left and right of the vaginal opening that secrete mucus to provide vaginal lubrication.

Biofeedback. Biofeedback training is a nonmedical treatment that helps people improve their health by taking conscious control of their muscles using real-time body signals. Physical therapists use biofeedback to help retrain the pelvic floor muscles.

Cesarean Section (C-Section). A Cesarean section is a major abdominal surgery in which incisions are made through the mother's abdomen and uterus to deliver her child.

Chakra. Chakras are force centers that pulsate subtle energy. Seven major chakras are believed to exist within the body.

Chronic Pelvic Pain. A pelvic pain condition that persists for longer than three months. It is poorly understood and many times requires a multidisciplinary approach for successful treatment.

Clitoris. The clitoris, a female sex organ, is a multiplanar and three-dimensional structure and reaches deep within the female pelvis. It is neither flat, nor pointed nor straight but expansive and deeply connected to the vaginal wall, pubic bone, urethra and PFMs.

Clitoral Hood. This is a fold of skin that protects the glans of the clitoris. The clitoral hood should move freely and without pain.

Coccyx. This bone is found above the anus and in between the gluteal muscles.

Coccyxdynia or Coccygodynia. Pain in the area of the tailbone and its associated structures.

Connective Tissue Rolling (Skin Rolling). A type of massage that is superficial in nature and can be performed on any part of the body, including but not limited to, the abdomen, thighs, buttocks and lower back.

Crystal Wand. S-shaped tools that helps to reach deep PFMs trigger points. The crystal wand can also be used for PFMs massaging. Do not press too hard into the PFMs; this can potentially cause harm and injury.

Daily Voiding Log. A diary that helps you keep track of bowel and bladder habits. This tool allows you to quantify urge, leaking and eating and drinking habits.

Diastasis Recti. A separation of rectus abdominis muscle at its connective tissue the linea alba. Diastasis recti separation has been correlated with pelvic pain, abdominal trigger points, incontinence and organ prolapse.

Dilator. A medical instrument used to stretch and expand the vaginal opening. Dilators are also used for intravaginal and intrarectal massage of the pelvic floor muscles. Many times, dilators are also used for trigger point release therapy.

Dyspareunia. Painful sexual intercourse which can occur for many reasons including medical or psychological. Dyspareunia is almost always reported by women, but this problem can also occur in men.

Episiotomy. An episiotomy is a surgical incision made at the perineum to enlarge the vagina. This incision can be midline or medial-lateral. It is a common cause of sexual pain and can cause scar tissue in the perineum.

Fascia. Fascia is the soft tissue glue that holds the body together. It permeates the entire body, surrounding muscles, organs, nerves, blood vessels and other visceral structures. Fascia helps maintain structural integrity, provides support and protection, and acts as a shock absorber.

Fibromyalgia. A medical disorder that causes widespread body pain exacerbated by gentle touch. Additional symptoms include fatigue, sleep disturbance, and joint stiffness. This condition can also affect the respiratory, digestive and other body systems.

Glans of the Clitoris. This is an extension of the body of the clitoris (internal clitoris) and is partly on the outside.

Gluteus Medius. This is a gluteal muscle that is under the gluteus maximus and can be found to the outside of the butt cheek near the top of the hip bone. This muscle can refer pain to perineum, labia, hip, posterior thigh and sit bone. It can also refer sciatica-like symptoms.

Greater Trochanter of the Femur. This is not a muscle but a very important area that tends to have trigger points and can be a big source of pelvic and hip pain. Many of the posterior hip muscles insert into this bone and it is necessary to reduce or eliminate pain in this area.

Hart's Line. The edge of the vulvar vestibule frequently examined for pain. The Q-tip test is the gold standard for determining abnormalities and pain in this area.

Hymenectomy. A surgical operation to remove the hymen.

Incontinence. Any involuntary leakage or loss of urine.

Interstitial Cystitis. Interstitial cystitis/painful bladder syndrome (IC/PBS) is a bladder disease characterized by painful urination, urinary frequency and urgency, and pressure in the bladder and/or pelvis. IC can also cause spasms and trigger points in the pelvic floor muscles.

Intra-Abdominal Pressure. Pressure within the abdominal cavity.

Iliac Crest Line. This is not a muscle but an area where many muscles live. It is the top of hip crest.

Ischioanal Fossa. A wedge-shaped space found on either side of the anal canal. This fossa houses important structures such as the pudendal canal, pudendal nerve, pudendal artery and pudendal vein. Dysfunction in the ischioanal fossa can lead to deep pelvic pain and pain with pressure, such as sitting.

"Just in Case" (JIC) Urination. This occurs when one urinates out of habit instead of waiting for a proper bladder signal or urinating when the bladder is full. JIC urination is dysfunctional and needs to be eliminated to properly re-train the bladder back to health.

Kegel. An exercise named after Dr. Arnold Kegel that consists of contracting and relaxing the pelvic floor muscles.

L1-L5. L1 through L5 represent the five lumbar spinal vertebrae. The lumbar vertebrae are found between the thoracic and sacral vertebrae in the spinal column. Many times, women with pelvic pain will have some kind of associated dysfunction with L5 and the lumbar spine.

Labia. The labia majora are the outer vaginal lips and are composed mostly of skin and adipose (fat) tissue. Protection is their main function. The labia minora are the inner vaginal lips on either side of the vaginal opening. The clitoris is the area where labia minora meet superiorly.

Laparoscopic Procedure. Surgical operation commonly performed within the abdominal or pelvic cavities using small keyhole-size incisions.

Levator Ani Muscles. The muscles that make up the pelvic floor.

Levator Ani Spasms. Involuntary contractions of the pelvic floor muscles that can lead to pain with sexual intercourse, sitting or other simple daily activities.

Levator Ani Syndrome. Consists of pain, pressure, discomfort or deep dull ache in the vagina and rectum, including the sacrum and coccyx. Levator ani syndrome can also cause burning or radiating pain into the thighs and buttocks. Pain with sitting and defecation are common complaints. Many times the pelvic floor muscles are in spasms and have multiple trigger points in them.

Lichen Sclerosus. An uncommon disease which may cause white patches or scarring on and around genital skin.

Marinoff Scale. A scale that quantifies pain as it relates to sexual intercourse.

Mons Pubis. It is the fatty tissue lying above the pubic bone of adult women.

Muscle Golgi Tendon Apparatus. The Golgi tendon organ is a proprioceptive sensory receptor located at the insertion of skeletal muscle fibers. This receptor monitors tension in the muscles. If there is excessive tension, the Golgi tendon will send a message that tells the muscle to relax.

Muscle Spindles. These are sensory receptors located within the belly of a muscle that detect changes in the length of the muscle fiber. This detection plays an important role in regulating muscle contraction. This information also helps the brain to determine the position of the body.

Myofascial Release. This is a connective tissue hands-on therapy for the treatment of muscle pain and immobility.

Myomectomy. Refers to the surgical removal of uterine fibroids.

Nantes Criteria. A clinical tool and assessment to facilitate the diagnosis of Pudendal Nerve Neuralgia (PNN) by Pudendal Nerve Entrapment (PNE). The Nantes criteria for PNN by PNE include:

1. Pain in the distribution of the pudendal nerve;
2. Pain that is increased and predominantly found with sitting;
3. The pain does not keep the patient awake at night;
4. No objective sensory impairments are found; and
5. Administration of a pudendal block relieves pain.

Neuropathic Pain. Neuropathic pain is not related to the activation of pain receptor cells in any part of the body. This type of pain is produced by a change or injury to neurological structure or function of the tissue.

Neutral Spine (NS). Neutral spine is the natural position of the spine when all the parts of the spine, cervical, thoracic and lumbar, are in excellent alignment.

Obturator Internus Muscle. The obturator internus muscle is found within the pelvis and within the hip-joint. This muscle helps to externally rotate the leg, extend the thigh and abduct the flexed thigh. It also helps to stabilize femoral head in the acetabulum. This muscle can cause sexual pain, hip pain and/or a deep ache in the pelvis. The obturator internus can refer pain to anywhere within the pelvic girdle. This muscle can be accessed through the vagina and rectum and can frequently have spasms and trigger points causing sexual and pelvic pain.

Pelvic Floor Muscle Dysfunction. Abnormal or impaired function of the pelvic floor muscles.

Pelvic Floor Muscle Hypertonicity. Muscular hypertonicity is a disorder in which muscles continually receive a message to tighten and to contract. This causes excessive stiffness or tightness and interferes with their normal function.

Pelvic Floor Muscle Incoordination. A lack of normal and harmonious muscle action in the pelvic floor muscles.

Pelvic Floor Muscle Spasm. Involuntary contraction of a pelvic floor muscle.

Pelvic Girdle. The muscles, bones and ligaments of the pelvic and hip region.

Pelvic Release. A lengthening release of the pelvic floor muscles that can be performed with either inhalation or exhalation.

Perineal Body. The central area between the rectum and the vagina in the perineum. It is also the area where most of the pelvic floor muscles are attached.

Perineal Tearing. Tears to the perineum (the area between the genitalia and anus) that can cause damage to the anal sphincter causing fecal incontinence, urgency, pain during intercourse or other problems.

Perineal Tears in Degrees. Tears are rated from 1st to 4th Degree. 1st Degree is tearing of the vaginal mucosa skin at or around the perineal body. 2nd Degree is tearing vaginal mucosa and submucosa through the pelvic floor muscles. 3rd Degree is tearing of the 1st and 2nd Degree tissues and the external sphincter. 4th Degree is all of the above levels of tearing plus the internal sphincter and the lining of the rectum.

Perineum. The diamond-shaped area between the legs that houses muscles and rectum, and in females, includes the vagina. This can also refer to both the superficial or deep structures in this region.

Persistent Genital Arousal Disorder (PGAD). Spontaneous, persistent, and uncontrollable genital arousal without sexual contact or thoughts.

Piriformis Syndrome. A disorder that occurs when the sciatic nerve is compressed, pinched or irritated by the piriformis muscle. This compression can cause pain, tingling and numbness in the buttocks and along the sciatic nerve path.

Prolapse. This term is used for organs that protrude through the vagina. This condition makes the organ drop into the vagina causing pelvic floor muscle weakness. The uterus, rectum, bladder or urethra can prolapse into the vagina.

Psoas Muscle. This is deep muscle that cannot be seen from the outside of the body. It comes from lumbar spine and inserts into the top of the leg bone. This muscle can be a source of pelvic pain and many times has trigger points in it that refer pain to the hip, low back and vulvar-vaginal area

Pubic Bone. This bone forms the anterior aspect of the pelvis and hip bones.

Pudendal Nerve. This nerve arises from the ventral rami of nerve roots S2 to S4 and from the pudendal nerve trunk. The pudendal nerve is a mix nerve with sensory, motor and autonomic fibers. It has three terminal branches that include dorsal nerve of the clitoris, perineal branch and inferior rectal branch.
The pudendal nerve is the main nerve of the perineum and supplies the PFMs, vagina, urethra, skin of labia, external anal sphincter, urethral sphincter, anal canal, anal skin, clitoris and sensory to the lower vagina.

Pudendal Nerve Canal (PNC) Syndrome. An issue of the pudendal nerve as it travels within Alcock's canal and becomes irritated, compressed or entrapped.

Pudendal Nerve Entrapment (PNE). Pudendal nerve entrapment is a source of chronic pain in which the pudendal nerve is entrapped or compressed via muscles, fascia and/or ligaments.

Pudendal Nerve Neuralgia (PNN). A shooting, stabbing and knife-like pain that can occur anywhere in the distribution of the pudendal nerve.

Quadratus Lumborum. This muscle can be found posterior in between the lower ribs and the top of the hip bone but lateral to the paraspinal muscles. Once you are in this area you have to press in toward the spine to find the trigger point. This muscle can be a big pelvic pain generator and must be addressed.

Rectus Abdominis. This is the six-pack abdominal muscle; it runs from below the breast bone to the pubic bone. There are two sides, one to the right of the belly button and one to the left that are connective via the linea alba. A separation of this muscle at the linea alba is called diastasis recti.

Resting Baseline of the Pelvic Floor Muscles. It is the biofeedback readout that reports the activity of the muscles while a person is at rest. Normally, most individuals have low resting baselines; however, women suffering from sexual pain usually have elevated resting baselines.

Reverse Kegel. This exercise is an elongation and relaxation exercise for the PFMs.

S2-S5. S2 through S5 are vertebrae of the sacral spine. The sacral spine is below the lumbar spine and is located at the base of the spine.

Sacroiliac Joint (SI Joint). This is the joint between the sacrum and the ilium hip bone joined by ligaments. It is a strong, weight-bearing joint that can generate extreme discomfort for women with chronic pelvic pain.

Sacrospinous Ligament. A ligament that is attached to the ischial spine, sacrum and coccyx.

Sacrotuberous Ligament. A ligament that runs from the ischial tuberosity (sit bone) to the sacrum.

Sacrum. The sacrum is a triangular bone at the base of the spine where it is inserted like a wedge between the two hip bones. Its upper edge connects to the last lumbar vertebra, and its bottom connects with the coccyx (tailbone). The sacral nerves exit through small holes in the sacrum.

Scar. A scar is part of the natural healing process of wound repair in the skin and other tissues of the body.

Sit Bones. Also called ischial tuberosity, sit bones are the bones that we sit on. These bones have surrounding fascia that are intimately connected with the gluteal and hip muscles. Many times women suffering from pelvic pain experience pain at these bones. Many times the gluteal muscles, adductor muscles, PFMs and PNN can refer pain to the sit bones. An exhaustive investigation will have to be done to find out exactly why there is sit bone pain.

Skin Rolling. Also know as connective tissue rolling, this is a type of massage used for releasing and clearing barriers, and fascial restrictions and trigger points in muscles.

Strain-Counterstrain. A technique invented by Dr. Lawrence Jones, where muscles are put in a position of maximum contraction for 90 seconds, allowing the muscle to rest. This technique relieves pain and results in better muscle function.

Suprapubic Abdominal Muscles. This is an area, not really a muscle. This is the abdominal muscle area that resides on top of the pubic bone and is frequently loaded with trigger points that contribute to bladder symptoms including urgency.

Tendinous Arch of the Levator Ani. A thickened portion of the obturator fascia where some of the levator ani muscles originate. This fascia can be painful to the touch. Let an experienced PT show you how to correctly release this fascia.

Tension Release Breathing (TRB). A breathing technique coined by author Isa Herrera using mind/body connection to release pain and tension of a painful muscle. The individual inhales into the painful body part while thinking about collecting her pain as she inhales. Then the individual exhales and visualizes the pain leaving her body. This type of breathing should be performed for 5 breaths.

Tinel Sign. A test that detects irritated nerves and is performed by gently tapping on the nerve to elicit a sensation of pins and needles in the distribution of the nerve.

Transversus Abdominis Muscle. This is the deepest abdominal muscle and it has an intimate relationship with the PFMs.

Urge Control and Suppression Techniques. These are tools and techniques that help to delay voiding and can buy you time until you find a bathroom. They work to retrain the bladder back to health.

Urgency or Frequency of Urination. Frequent urination or urgency of urination without an increase in the total urine held in the bladder. This condition may result from infections, a small bladder capacity, other structural abnormalities, from food irritants, or trigger points.

Urinary Tract Infections (UTI). An infection that affects part of the urinary tract which includes the bladder, kidneys or tubes that connect the bladder to the kidneys. Most UTI are bladder infections. Symptoms of UTI can include painful urination, frequent urination or urge to urinate.

Vaginismus. A condition in which the pelvic floor muscles go into spasms or tense suddenly, making penetration impossible. Women who suffer from this condition experience difficulty or pain with sexual relations, problems with inserting tampons, or penetration involved with gynecological examinations. This condition can be a result of an involuntary muscular reflex.

Vestibulectomy. Surgical removal of extremely painful tissue of the vaginal vestibule.

Vestibulodynia. Also known as vestibulitis, this is pain and discomfort in the vulva vestibule area.

Vulva. The vulva is part of the external genitalia of a woman. This area surrounds the opening of the vagina.

Vulvar Biopsy. A biopsy performed under local anesthesia to obtain a small sample of vulvar epithelium for examination.

Vulvodynia, Provoked. A type of vulvodynia that occurs with direct contact with the vulva.

Vulvodynia, Unprovoked. A type of vulvodynia that causes vulvar pain, burning, and discomfort without direct contact to the vulva area.

Young Living Oils. An online company that sells therapeutic grade essentials oils. To buy oils from this company you need to have a subscriber number. Use mine — #1422496 — to register. To get the best prices, register as a wholesaler.

Bibliography

Abbott, J. (2009). Gynecological indications for the use of botulinum toxin in women with chronic pelvic pain. *Toxicon.* 2009 Oct; 54(5):647-53. Epub 2009 Mar 3.

Abbott, J., Jarvis, S., Lyons, S., Thomson, A., & Vancaille, T. (2006). Botulinum toxin type A for chronic pain and pelvic floor spasm in women: a randomized controlled trial. *Obstetrics & Gynecology,* 108(4), 915-923.

Abraham, K. (2002). A special update on chronic pelvic pain from the conference: Chronic pelvic pain: Pathogenic mechanisms, treatment, innovations, and research implications. *Journal of the Section on Women's Health,* 26(3), 9-12.

Albert, H., Godskesen, M., Westergaard, J. (1999). Evaluation of clinical tests used in classification procedures in pregnancy-related pelvic joint pain. *European Spine Journal,* 9(2) 161-166.

Arvigo, Rosita, and Epstein, Nadine. (2001). *Rainforest Remedies: The Maya Way to Heal Your Body & Replenish Your Soul.* New York, NY: Harper Collins Publishers.

Barral, Jean-Pierre. (1993). *Urogenital Manipulation.* Seattle, WA: Eastland Press.

Barral, Jean-Pierre. (1989). *Visceral Manipulation.* Seattle, WA: Eastland Press.

Barral, Jean-Pierre and Mercier, Pierre. (2005). *Visceral Manipulation, Revised Edition.* Seattle, WA: Eastland Press.

Barral, Jean-Pierre. (2007). *Visceral Manipulation II (Revised Edtion)*. Seattle WA: Eastland Press.

Barral, Jean-Pierre, and Kuchera, Michael L. (2007). *Visceral and Obstetric Osteopathy*. Edinburgh, England: Churchill Livingstone.

Barral, Jean-Pierre, DO, Wetzler, Gail, RPT, Ahern, Dee, RPT, Grant, Lisa Brady, DC. (2005). *Visceral Manipulation: Abdomen 2 Study Guide*. West Palm Beach, FL: The Barral Institute.

Barral, Jean-Pierre, DO, Wetzler, Gail, RPT. (2005). *Visceral Manipulation: Abdomen 1 Study Guide*. West Palm Beach, FL: The Barral Institute.

Beco, Jacques. (2001).Relevant Anatomy of Pudendal Nerve and Etiological Factors of Pudendal Neuropathies Retrieved February 18, 2014 from http://www. perineology.com/files/ics-glasgow-anatomy.pdf.

Bergeron, S., et al. (2001). Vulvar vestibular syndrome: Reliability of diagnosis and evaluation of current diagnostic criteria. *Obstet Gynecol*. Vol. 98, 45-51.

Bergeron, S., Binik, Y. M., Khalifé, S., Pagidas, K., & Glazer, H. I. (2001). Vulvar vestibular syndrome: Rehabilitation of diagnosis and evaluation of current diagnostic criteria. *Obstetrics & Gynecology*, 98(1), 45-51.

Berghmans, L. C., Hendriks, H. J., Bo, K., Hay-Smith, E. J., de Bie, R. A., & van Waalwijk van Doorn, E. S. (1998). Conservative treatment of stress urinary incontinence in women: A systematic review of randomized clinical trials. *British Journal of Urology*, 82(2), 181-91.

Berghmans, L., Frederiks, C., de Bie, R., Weil, E., Smeets, L., van Waalwijk van Doorn, E, et al. (1996). Efficacy of biofeedback, when included with pelvic floor muscle exercise treatment, for genuine stress incontinence. *Neurology and Urody-namics*,15(1), 37-52.

Block, Jennifer. (2007). *Pushed. The Painful Truth About Childbirth and Modern Maternity Care*. Cambridge, MA: Da Capo Press.

Bo, Kari, Berghmans, Bary, Morkved, Siv, Van Kampen, Marijke.(2007). *Evidence-Based Physical Therapy for the Pelvic Floor*. London: Churchill Livingstone, Elselvier Health Sciences.

Bo, K., & Sherburn, M. (2005). Evaluation of female pelvic floor muscle function and strength. *Physical Therapy*, 85(3), 269-282.

Borello-France, D., Zyczynski, H., Downey, P, Rause, C. & Wister, J. (2006). Effect of pelvic-floor muscle exercise position on continence and quality-of-life outcomes in women with stress urinary incontinence. *Physical Therapy*, 86(7), 974-986.

Bouchez, Colette. (2001). *The V Zone: A Woman's Guide to Intimate Health Care*. New York, NY: Fireside.

Butler, D. S. (2004). *Mobilisation of the Nervous System*. Edinborough: Churchill Livingston.

Calais-Germain, Blandine. (2003). *The Female Pelvis: Anatomy & Exercises*. Seattle, WA: Eastland Press.

Calais-Germain, Blandine. (2005). *Anatomy of Breathing*. Seattle, WA: Eastland Press.

Calleja-Agius J, Brincat MP. (2009). Urogenital atrophy. *Climacteric*. Apr 22, pp. 1-7.

Carriere, Neate, and Feldt, Cynthia Markel. (2006). *The Pelvic Floor*. Stuttgart, Germany: Georg Thieme Verlag.

Cauthery, Dr. Philip, Stanway, Dr. Andrew, and Stanway, Dr. Penny. (1983). *The Complete Book of Love and Sex*. Great Britain: Century Publishing Co. Ltd.

Chaitow, Leon, Lovegrove Jones, Ruth. (2012). *Chronic Pelvic Pain and Dysfunction: Practical Physical Medicine*. London: Churchill Livingstone, Elselvier Health Sciences.

Chaitow, Leon. (2006). *Muscle Energy Techniques*. London: Churchill Livingstone,Elselvier Health Sciences.

Chaitow, Leon. (2007). *Positional Release Techniques*. London: Churchill Livingstone,Elselvier Health Sciences.

Chu, K. K., Chen, F. P., Chang, S. D., & Soong, Y. K. (1995). Laparoscopic presacral neurectomy in the treatment of dysmenorrhea. *Diagnostic and Therapeutic Endoscopy*, 1, 223-225.

Coccydynia. (n.d.). In Wikipedia. Retrieved March 10, 2014 from http://en.wikipedia.org/wiki/Coccydynia.

D'Amborosio, Kerry J, Roth, George B. (1997). *Positional Release Therapy, Assessment and Treatment of Musculoskeletal Dysfunction*. St. Louis, MO: Mosby.

Davies, Clair and Amber Davies. (2004). *The Trigger Point Therapy Workbook: Your Self-Treatment Guide for Pain Relief*. Oakland, CA: New Harbinger Publications.

Davis, Martha, Ph.D, Robbins-Eshelman, Elizabeth, M.S.W., and McKay, Matthew, Ph.D. (2000). *The Relaxation and Stress Reduction Workbook*. New York, NY: MJM Books.

Dell, JR, Mokrzycki, ML, Jayne, CJ. (2009). Differentiating interstitial cystitis from similar conditions commonly seen in gynecologic practice. *Eur J Obstet Gynecol Reprod Biol*. Apr 29.

Derry, DE. (1907). Pelvic muscles and fasciae. *Journal of Anatomy and Physiology*,42:107-11.

Drake, Richard L., Vogl, A. Wayne, Mitchell, Adam W.M., Tibbitts, Richard M., Richardson, Paul E. (2008). *Gray's Atlas of Anatomy*. London: Churchill Livingstone, Elselvier Health Sciences.

Dul, Jan and Weerdmeester, Bernard. (2001). *Ergonomics for Beginners: A Quick Reference Guide. Second Edition*. London: Taylor & Francis.

Dumoulin, C., Lemieux, M., Bourbonnais, D., Gravel, D., Bravo, G. & Morin, M. (2004). Physiotherapy for persistent postnatal stress urinary incontinence: a randomized controlled trial. *Obstetrics & Gynecology*, 104(3), 504-510.

Dye, J. (2004). Fertility of American Women: June 2004. *Current Population Report*, December 2005, 1-14.

Ehrstrom S, Kornfeld D, Rylander E, Bohm-Starke N. (2009). Chronic stress in women with localized provoked vulvodynia. *J Psychosom Obstet Gynaecol*. March Vol. 30(1), pp. 73-9.

Epstein, Abby, and Lake, Ricki. (2009). *Your Best Birth*. New York, NY: Hachette Book Group.

Fanucci E, Manenti G, Ursone A, Fusco N, Mylonakou I, D'Urso S, Simonetti G. (2009). Role of interventional radiology in pudendal neuralgia: a description of techniques and review of the literature. *Radiol Med.* Mar 10.

Fisher, K. & Riolo, L. (2004). Evidence in practice. *American Physical Therapy Association Inc.* Retrieved June 12, 2008 from http://www.thefreelibrary.com/ evidence+in+practice-a0120610455.com.

FitzGerald, M.P. & Kotarinos, R. (2003). Rehabilitation of the short pelvic floor. I: Background and patient evaluation. *International Urogynecological Journal,* 14(4), 261-268.

FitzGerald, M.P. & Kotarinos, R. (2003). Rehabilitation of the short pelvic floor, II: Treatment of the patient with the short pelvic floor. *International Urogynecological Journal,* 14 (4), 269-275.

Foye, Patrick, & Buttacci, Charles. (2012). Coccyx Pain. *In Medscape.* Retrieved March 10, 2014 from http://emedicine.medscape.com/article/309486-overview#aw2aab6b2b2.

Foye, Patrick, & Buttacci, Charles. (2012). Coccyx Pain Treatment & Management. *In Medscape.* Retrieved March 12, 2014 from http://emedicine.medscape.com/article/309486-treatment#aw2aab6b6b3.

Franklin, Eric. (2002). *Pelvic Power: Mind/Body Exercises for Strength, Flexibility, Posture, and Balance.* Hightstown, NJ: Princeton Book Company.

Gerwin, R., Dommerholt, J., & Shah, J. (2004). An explanation of simons' integrated hypothesis of trigger point formation. *Current Science Inc.,* 8, 468-475.

Glazer, H., & MacConkey, D. (1996). Functional rehabilitation of pelvic floor muscles: A challenge to tradition. Urologic Nursing, 16, 68-9. Retrieved May 25, 2008 from http://www.vulvodynia.com/fropfm.htm.

Goldberg, Roger. (2003). *Ever Since I Had My Baby: Understanding, Treating, and Preventing the Most Common Physical Aftereffects of Pregnancy and Childbirth.* New York, NY: Three Rivers Press.

Goldfinger C, Pukall CF, Gentilcore-Saulnier E, McLean L, Chamberlain S. (2009). A prospective study of pelvic floor physical therapy: Pain and psycho-sexual outcomes in provoked vestibulodynia. *J Sex Med.* April 28.

Goldstein, A. (2008). Vulvodynia (CME). *J Sex Med.* 2008 Jan;5 (1):5-15 18173761. Retrieved December 12, 2008, from http://lib.bioinfo.pl/auth:Goldstein,AT.

Goldstein, A. (2007). New diagnosis for vestibular pain and redness: Don't get lumped in a general category again! *OurGyn.* Retrieved February 12, 2009, from http://www.ourgyn.com.

Goldstein, A. (2007). Vaginal pain and itching with no known cause? *OurGyn.* Retrieved February 21, 2009, from http://www.ourgyn.com.

Goldstein, A. (2007). 14 different treatments for vulvar vestibulitis syndrome. *OurGyn.* Retrieved May 23, 2008 from http://www.ourgyn.com/content/index. php?option=com_content&task=view&id=18&Itemid=66.

Goldfinger, S. (2007). Gas and bloating. *UpToDate.* Retrieved July 11, 2008, from http://www.uptodate.com/patients/content/topic.do?topicKey=~ S6QjVerp-W9eT4.

Gustafson, KJ, Zelkovic, PF, Feng, AH, Draper, CE, Bodner, DR, Grill, WM. (2005). Fascicular anatomy and surgical access of the human pudendal nerve. *World J Urol*. 2005 Dec; 23(6):411-8. Epub 2005 Dec 7. Retrieved February 10, 2014 from http://www.ncbi.nlm.nih.gov/pubmed/16333625.

Haefner, H., Collins, M., Davis, G., Edwards, L., Foster, D., Hartmann, E., et al (2005). The Vulvodynia Guideline. *Journal of Lower Genital Tract Disease*, 9(1), 40-51.

Harlow, B., & Stewart, E. (2003). A population-based assessment of chronic unexplained vulvar pain: Have we underestimated the prevalence of vulvodynia? *Journal of the American Medical Women's Association*, 58(2), 82-87.

Haslam, Jeanette, and Laycock, Jo. (2002). *Therapeutic Management of Incontinence and Pelvic Pain. Second Edition*. London, England: Springer-Verlag.

Hay, Louise L. (1999). *You Can Heal Your Life*. Carlsbad, CA: Hay House Inc.

Hopwood, Val, and Lovesey, Maureen, and Mokone, Sara. (1997). *Acupuncture & Related Techniques in Physical Therapy*. Edinburgh, England: Churchill Livingstone.

Hruby S, Ebmer J, Dellon AL, Aszmann, OC. (2005). Anatomy of the pudendal nerve at the urogenital diaphragm: A new critical site for nerve entrapment, *Urology*, 66: 949-952.

Hulme, Janet A. (1997). *Beyond Kegels. Second Edition*. Missoula, MT: Phoenix Publishing Co.

Hutcherson, Hilda. (2002). *What Your Mother Never Told You About S-e-x*. New York, NY: Berkley Publishing Group.

Jones, L. H., Kusunose, R. H. & Goering, E. K. (1995). *Jones Strain-Counterstrain*. Boise, ID: Jones Strain-Counterstrain Inc.

Kabatt-Zin, Jon. (2005). *Coming to Our Senses*. New York, NY: Hyperion.

Katz, Ditza and Ross Lynn Tabisel. (2005). *Private Pain: Understanding Vaginismus & Dyspareunia. Second Edition*. Canada: Katz-Tabi Publications.

Kavaler, Elizabeth. (2006). *A Seat on the Aisle, Please: The Essential Guide to Urinary Tract Problems in Women*. New York, NY: Copernicus Books.

Kellogg-Spadt, S., & Albaugh, J. (2002). Intimacy and bladder pain: helping women reclaim sexuality. *Urologic Nursing*, 22(5), 355-56.

Kellogg-Spadt, S., & Giordano, J. (2002). Vulvar Vestibulitis and Sexual Pain. *The Female Patient*, 27, 51-53.

Klein, M., & Robbins, R. (1998). *Let Me Count the Ways: Discovering Great Sex Without Intercourse*. New York, NY: Penguin Putnam Inc.

KMom (2003). Pelvic pain (Symphysis publis dysfunction). Retrieved August 14, 2008, from http://www.plus-size-pregnancy.org/pubicpain.htm.

Lachowsky M, Nappi R. (2009). The effects of estrogen on urogenital health. *Maturitas*. April 30.

Lee, R. B., Stone, K., Magelssen, D., Belts, R. P., & Benson, W. L. (1986). Presacral neurectomy for chronic pelvic pain. *Obstetrics & Gynecology*, 68, 517-521. Retrieved April 17, 2008, from http://www.greenjournal.org/cgi/content/abstract/68/4/517.

Levin-Gervasi, Stephanie. (1995). *The Back Pain Sourcebook.* Los Angeles, CA: Lowell House.

Magee, David J. (2002). *Orthopedic Physical Assessment.* Philadelphia, PA: Saunders Publications.

Maigne, Jean-Yves. (2002). *Management of Common Coccygodynia.* Retrieved February1, 2014 from http://www.coccyx.org/medabs/maigne6.htm .

Makichen, Walter. (2005). *Spirit Babies. How to Communicate with the Child You're Meant to Have.* New York, NY: Bantam Dell.

Manheim, Carol. (2001). *The Myofascial Release Manual. Third Edition.* Thorofare, NJ: Slack Inc.

Mercier, Patricia. (2007). *The Chakra Bible.* New York, NY: Sterling Publishing.

Miller, P., Forstein, D. & Styles, S. (2008). Effect of short-term diet and exercise on hormone levels and menses in obese, infertile women. *Journal of Reproductive Medicine*, 53(5), 315-319.

Mojay, Gabriel. (1997). *Aromatherapy for Healing the Spirit: Restoring Emotional and Mental Balance with Essential Oils.* Rochester, Vermont: Healing Arts Press.

Moldwin, R. (2000). *The Interstitial Cystitis Survival Guide: Your Guide to the Latest Treatment Options and Coping Strategies*. Oakland, CA: New Harbinger Publications.

Morkved, S., Bo, K. & Fjortoft, T. (2002). Effect of adding biofeedback to pelvic floor muscle training to treat urodynamic stress incontinence. *Obstetrics & Gynecology*,100(4), 730-739.

Myers, Thomas W. (2001). *Anatomy Trains. Myofascial Meridians and Movement Therapists*. Edinburgh, England: Churchill Livingstone.

Netter, Frank H. (1989). *Atlas of Human Anatomy*. Teterboro, NJ: Icon Learning Systems.

Neumann, Donald A. (2002). *Kinesiology of the Musculoskeletal System: Foundations or Physical Rehabilitation*. St. Louis: Mosby Inc.

Newman, D. (2008). Understanding electrical stimulation as a treatment for incontinence. *Seekwellness*. Retrieved January 14, 2009, from http://www.seekwellness.com/incontinence/electric_stim.htm.

Noble, Elizabeth. (1995). *Essential Exercises for the Childbearing Year*. Harwich, MA: New Life Images.

Paoletti, Serge. (2006*). The Fasciae Anatomy, Dysfunction and Treatment*. Seattle, WA: Eastland Press

Pelvic Health Solutions: Active Pudendal Nerve Gliding. Retrieved February 1, 2014 from http://www.pelvichealthsolutions.ca/for-the-patient/pudendal-nerve-irritation/neural-tension/.

Prendergast, S., & Weiss, J. (2003). Screening for musculoskeletal causes of pelvic pain. *Clinical Obstetrics & Gynecology*, 46(4), 1-10.

Prendergast, S. How do I know if I have PN or PNE? *Pelvic Health and Rehabilitation Center.* Retrieved January 14, 2014 http://www.pelvicpainrehab.com/pelvic-pain/726/how-do-i-know-if-i-have-pn-or-pne/

Rao, S. (2004). Diagnosis and management of fecal incontinence. *The American Journal of Gastroenterology*, 99(8), 1585-1604.

Rogers, Rebecca G, Janet Yagoda Shagam and Shelley Kleinschmidt. (2006). *Regaining Bladder Control: What Every Woman Needs to Know.* New York, NY: Prometheus Books.

Sahrmann, A. Shirley. (2002). *Diagnosis and Treatment of Movement Impairment Syndromes.* St. Louis, Mosby Inc.

Sapsford, R., & Hodges, P. (2001). Contraction of the pelvic floor muscles during abdominal maneuvers. *Archives of Physical Medicine and Rehabilitation*, 82(8), 1081-8.

Sapsford Aua, Ruth et al. (1998). *Women's Health: A Textbook for Physiotherapists.* New York: WB Saunders Company Ltd.

Sapsford, R. (2001). "Contraction of the pelvic floor muscles during abdominal maneuvers." Abstract: *Arch Phys Med Rehabil.* Vol. 81, 1081-8.

Schnaubet, Kurt. (1999). *Medical Aromatherapy. Healing with Essential Oils.* Berkely, CA: Frog, Ltd.

Shamliyan, T., Kane, R., Wyman, J. & Wilt, T. (2008). Systematic review: randomized, controlled trials of nonsurgical treatments for urinary incontinence in women. *Annals of Internal Medicine,* 148(6), 459-473.

Spadt-Kellogg, S.,et al. (2002). Vulvar vestibulitis and sexual pain: New insights. *The Female Patient.* Vol. 27, 51-53.

Spadt-Kellogg, Susan, et al. (2002). Intimacy and bladder pain: Helping women reclaim sexuality. *Urologic Nursing* Vol. 22:5, 355-56.

Spatafora, Denise. (2009). *Better Birth.* Hoboken, NJ: Wiley and Sons, Inc.

Steege JF, Zolnoun DA. (2009). Evaluation and treatment of dyspareunia. *Obstet Gynecol.* May 113(5), pp. 1124-36.

Stewart, Elizabeth G. and Paula Spencer. (2002). *The V Book: A Doctor's Guide to Complete Vulvovaginal Health.* New York, NY: Bantam Books.

Sutton KS, Pukall CF, Chamberlain S. (2009). Pain ratings, sensory thresholds, and psychosocial functioning in women with provoked vestibulodynia. *J Sex Marital Ther.* Vol. 35(4), pp. 262-81.

Tjaden, B., Schlaff, W. D., Kimball, A., & Rock, J. A. (1990). The efficacy of presacral neurectomy for the relief of midline dysmenorrhea. *Obstetrics & Gynecology,* 76, 89-91. Retrieved February 13, 2008, from http://www.greenjournal.org/cgi/content/abstract/76/1/89.

Tolle, Eckhart. (1999). *The Power of Now.* Vancouver, Canada: Namaste Publishing.

Wallace, Kathe and Holly Herman. (2006). *Female Pelvic Floor: Function, Dysfunction and Treatment. Level 2B.* The Prometheus Group: Secaucus, NJ, Nov 3-5 2006.

Wallace, Kathe and Holly Herman. (2007). *Female Pelvic Floor: Function, Dysfunction and Treatment. Level 3.* The Prometheus Group: New York, NY, May 4-6 2007.

Wallace, Kathe and Holly Herman. (2008). *Female Pelvic Floor: Function, Dysfunction and Treatment. Level 1.* The Prometheus Group: Hunter College, March 7-9 2008.

Weiss, J. (2000). Chronic pelvic pain and myofascial trigger points. *The Pain Clinic,* 13(6), 13-18.

Weiss, J. (2001). Pelvic floor myofascial trigger point: Manual therapy for interstitial cystitis and the urgency-frequency syndrome. *The Journal of Urology,* 166(6), 2226-2231.

Weiss, J. (2003). Pudendal nerve entrapment. Presented at the *International Pelvic Pain Society 10th Scientific Meeting of Chronic Pelvic Pain* in Alberta, Canada August 2003, 1-25.

Wetzler, Gail, PT. (2009). *Gynecologic Visceral Manipulation.* Alexandria, VA: American Physical Therapy Association.

Wise, D. & Anderson, R. (2003). *A Headache in the Pelvis: A New Understanding and Treatment for Chronic Pelvic Pain Syndromes.* Occidental, CA: National Center for Pelvic Pain.

Index

H

hart's line 56-58, 380

hypertonicity 18, 158, 169, 383

I

incontinence 35, 60, 301-302, 306, 332, 335, 379-380, 384

incoordination 18, 383

interstitial cystitis 20, 26, 43-44, 49, 376, 380

ischial 293, 298, 387

K

kegel 44, 60-65, 72-75, 79-80, 83, 90-92, 157-158, 166, 178, 204, 239, 266, 323, 326, 328-330, 333, 345, 360, 372, 381, 386

knobble 255

L

labia 30, 38, 42, 47, 52, 54, 56-57, 180-182, 192, 195, 197-198, 208, 210-212, 292, 299-300, 302, 380-381, 385

laparoscopic procedure 381

latent trigger points 3 9-40

levator ani 34, 36, 38, 55, 161, 172, 174, 180, 189, 191-192, 306-307, 381-382, 388

lichen schlerosis 43, 50

Y

yoga 28, 58, 75, 79, 84, 89-90, 92-93, 95, 97, 100-104, 157, 166, 272, 304-305, 338

young living oils 179, 183-184, 390

young living oils registration number 390

Made in the USA
San Bernardino, CA
24 August 2014